Multiple Choice Questions in General Surgery

Kefah M. Mokbel MB, BS (London), FRCS (England)

Department of Academic Surgery
Imperial College School of Medicine
St Mary's Hospital
London

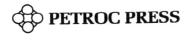 **PETROC PRESS**

Petroc Press, an imprint of LibraPharm Limited

Distributors

Plymbridge Distributors Limited, Plymbridge House, Estover Road, Plymouth PL6 7PZ, UK

Published in the United Kingdom by LibraPharm Limited, Gemini House, 162 Craven Road, Newbury, Berkshire RG14 5NR, UK

A catalogue record for this book is available from the British Library

ISBN 1 900603 10 1

Typeset by
Richard Powell Editorial and Production Services, Basingstoke, Hampshire
Printed and bound in the United Kingdom by
BPC Wheatons, Exeter

Contents

Part 2 Extended Matching Questions

Part 1
Multiple True–False Questions

1. Introduction

The multiple-choice question format as part of examinations has come to stay. In an essay assessment, the examiner has to search the paragraphs for relevant facts and opinion, and the examinee can hide behind the smoke screen of language. No such cover is provided by multiple-choice questions, which not only allow electronic marking but also provide a more comprehensive assessment of the candidate's knowledge and a fine stone to sharpen the knife of his or her knowledge.

The stimulus for writing this book came from the major changes in the postgraduate surgical examinations in the United Kingdom in 1995. The new examination leading to the award of Diploma of a Member (or an Associate Fellow) of the Royal College of Surgeons consists of three sections:

A. The first section consists of two multiple-choice question papers covering basic surgical sciences and clinical surgery.
B. The second section is a clinical section based on short cases.
C. The third section is the viva voce section. In this section, operative surgery and miscellaneous surgical topics are covered.

The MRCS (Eng) and AFRCS (Ed) written examinations comprise two multiple-choice papers. Paper 1 will test the candidate's knowledge of perioperative management, trauma, intensive care and neoplasia. Paper 2 will test the candidate's knowledge of the vascular and locomotor systems, head and neck, endocrine and paediatric disorders, breast disease, abdominal disorders, urology and transplantation. Questions will test the knowledge of basic science, clinical aspects, or a combination of both. Multiple true–false questions and extended matching type questions are used.

This book contains more than 440 multiple-choice questions (multiple true–false and extended matching types) covering basic sciences and clinical aspects of surgery in an integrated fashion. It also contains answers and teaching explanations. Although this book has been primarily written for candidates preparing for both MCQ papers of the MRCS and AFRCS (Ed) examinations, it will also be valuable to all other trainees preparing for postgraduate surgical examinations, general practitioners and senior medical students.

How to Use the Book

Each multiple true–false question consists of a main stem and five possible completions, each of which must be identified as true, false or don't know. Each extended-matching question's theme consists of six options (diagnoses, investigations or treatments) followed by a series of clinical presentations. For

4

each clinical presentation described, you must select the most likely option. Each correct response gains one mark and there is no penalty for an incorrect response. Good luck!

January, 1997 K.M.

2. Pre-operative Management

Q1 **The pre-operative management of a patient with obstructive jaundice includes:**

A. Intravenous mannitol infusion
B. Fresh frozen plasma
C. Intravenous broad-spectrum antimicrobials
D. Intravenous vitamin K
E. Endoscopic sphincterotomy of the sphincter of Oddi

Q2 **When a colectomy is performed on an insulin-dependent diabetic:**

A. The patient should be placed first on the operating list
B. The patient should receive one dose of medium-acting insulin on the morning of the operation
C. The postoperative insulin requirements will be less than normal daily requirements
D. The risk of wound infection will be approximately 3%
E. Blood glucose should be checked 1–2 hourly

Q3 **In a patient suffering from chronic obstructive airways disease, the following tests are useful in assessing the patient's fitness for anaesthesia:**

A. Spirometry
B. Carbon monoxide transfer factor
C. Arterial blood gas analysis
D. Pulmonary capillary wedge pressure
E. Peak expiratory flow rate

Q4 **In a patient who has had a myocardial infarction (MI) and requires a colectomy, the risk of reinfarction is:**

A. 15% if the operation is performed 2 months after MI
B. 4% if the operation is performed 7 months after MI
C. 15% if the operation is performed 5 months after MI
D. 35% if the operation is performed 1 month after MI
E. < 1% if the operation is performed 1 year later

Q5 **Diabetic ketoacidosis:**

A. May be triggered by infection
B. Has a higher mortality rate than hyperosmolar non-ketotic coma (HNC)
C. Is a recognised cause of cerebral oedema
D. Requires treatment with bicarbonate
E. Causes hyperkalaemia

6

Q6 The following operations are correctly paired with appropriate prophylactic antibiotics:

A. Laparoscopic cholecystectomy – Augmentin (Co-amoxiclav)
B. Appendicectomy (no perforation) – metronidazole 1 g PR
C. Colectomy – tetracycline
D. Gastrectomy – flucloxacillin
E. Total hip replacement – metronidazole

Q7 Bleeding due to the following disorders can be corrected with vitamin K:

A. Scurvy
B. Heparin over-anticoagulation
C. Warfarin over-anticoagulation
D. Haemophilia
E. Thrombocytopenia

Q8 Airflow limitation leads to a reduction in:

A. The forced expiratory volume in 1 second (FEV_1)
B. The ratio of FEV_1 to forced vital capacity (FVC)
C. Lung volumes
D. The ventilation perfusion ratio (i.e. $V/Q < 1$)
E. The peak expiratory flow rate (PEFR)

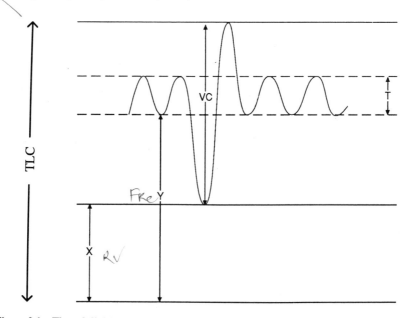

Figure 2.1 The subdivisions of the lung volume. T = resting tidal volume, TLC = total lung capacity, VC = vital capacity, X and Y = volumes

Q9   Figure 2.1 represents the subdivisions of the lung volume:

A. X is the functional residual capacity
B. Y is the expiratory reserve volume
C. TLC can be measured using a simple spirometer
D. A general anaesthetic increases Y
E. X is increased in a patient with emphysema

Q10   Captopril:

A. Completely inhibits renin
B. Is a recognised cause of neutropenia
C. Usually decreases serum potassium concentration
D. May cause proteinuria
E. Causes sodium and water retention

Q11   Drugs used in the treatment of cardiac failure include:

A. Enalpril
B. Indomethacin
C. Digoxin
D. Prednisolone
E. Dobutamine

Q12   With respect to anticoagulants:

A. Vitamin K reverses warfarin effects in 2 hours
B. Warfarin inhibits vitamin K epoxide reductase in the liver
C. Heparin is ineffective in patients with antithrombin III deficiency
D. Heparin's actions can be reversed with protamine sulphate
E. Laboratory monitoring is necessary when heparin is used in routine prophylaxis for deep vein thrombosis

Q13   In a patient with a sickle cell trait and a haemoglobin (Hb) level of 10 g/dl:

A. Sickling occurs if PaO_2 < 40 mmHg
B. Limb tourniquets are contraindicated
C. There is a homozygosity for the HbS gene
D. HbS concentration is approximately 1.5 g/dl
E. A pre-operative blood transfusion is necessary

Q14   A pre-operative blood pressure of 170/115 mmHg:

A. Increases the incidence of peri-operative stroke
B. Increases the incidence of peri-operative myocardial infarction
C. Should be treated prior to elective surgery
D. Is a contraindication to the use of isoflurane in anaesthesia
E. Reduces the risk of pulmonary embolism

8

Q15 A pacemaker should be inserted before surgery in the following conditions:

A. Stokes–Adams attacks
B. Complete heart block
C. Right bundle branch block with left axis deviation in an asymptomatic patient
D. Atrial fibrillation with a rate of 130 bpm
E. Atrial flutter with 2:1 block

Answers to Section 2

Q1
A. **True** – To reduce the incidence of hepatorenal syndrome (renal failure)
B. **True** – In severe hepatic impairment there is depletion of clotting factors
C. **True** – To reduce the incidence of septicaemia
D. **True** – To correct coagulopathy
E. **True** – To reduce the bilirubin level

Q2
A. **True** – If possible
B. **False** – All medium- and long-acting insulins should be stopped the night before
C. **False** – The insulin requirements will be increased by surgery
D. **False** – The risk will be much greater
E. **True** – An insulin sliding scale regimen (with 5% dextrose) is usually required until the patient starts oral feeding

Q3
A. **True** – e.g. FEV_1 and FVC
B. **False** – This measures the lung diffusion capacity
C. **True**
D. **False** – This is relevant to left ventricular failure. A Swan–Ganz catheter is necessary
E. **True**

Q4
A. **False** – The risk is 35%
B. **True**
C. **True**
D. **True**
E. **False** – The risk is approximately 3%

Q5
A. **True** – It may also be triggered by inadequate insulin therapy
B. **False** – HNC has a higher mortality rate
C. **True** – Treatment may cause rapid changes of plasma osmolarity precipitating cerebral oedema
D. **False** – Correction of water and electrolytes disturbance and insulin therapy are usually sufficient to correct acidosis
E. **True**

Q6
A. **True**
B. **True**
C. **False** – Antibiotics active against Gram-negative bacteria (e.g. *E. coli*) and anaerobes are required
D. **False** – Cefuroxime plus metronidazole may be used in prophylaxis
E. **False** – Flucloxacillin, cefuroxime or Augmentin may be used

Q7

A. **False** – Scurvy is due to vitamin C deficiency resulting in increased capillary fragility and bleeding

B. **False** – Protamine sulphate (1 mg for 100 units of heparin) or fresh frozen plasma can correct the over-anticoagulation

C. **True** – Factors II, VII, IX and X are vitamin K dependent

D. **False** – Factor VIII is not vitamin K dependent

E. **False** – Platelet transfusion is needed

Q8

A. **True**

B. **True**

C. **False** – Lung volumes are normal or increased

D. **True**

E. **True**

Q9

A. **False** – X is the residual volume

B. **False** – Y is the functional residual capacity (FRC)

C. **False** – This requires other techniques, e.g. helium dilution

D. **False** – As the subject lies down the diaphragm rises, thus reducing the FRC (Y)

E. **True**

Q10

A. **False** – It inhibits angiotensin converting enzymes

B. **True**

C. **False** – Hyperkalaemia may ensue

D. **True** – A true nephrotic syndrome is rarely seen

E. **False** – It increases sodium and water excretion

Q11

A. **True** – ACE inhibitors have been shown to prolong life in patients with chronic cardiac failure

B. **False** – This drug may induce cardiac failure by causing fluid retention

C. **True** – Digoxin is more effective in the presence of atrial fibrillation

D. **False** – Corticosteroids cause fluid retention

E. **True** – This inotropic agent increases contractility

Q12

A. **False** – It takes approximately 24 hours

B. **True** – This reduces the levels of clotting factors II, VII, IX and X

C. **True** – Heparin acts by enhancing antithrombin III

D. **True**

E. **False** – Prophylaxis dose is 5000 units twice a day (subcutaneously)

Q13
A. **True** – Hypoxia may cause sickling
B. **True** – Tourniquets may precipitate sickling
C. **False** – The patient is heterozygous for the HbS gene
D. **False** – 35% of total Hb is HbS, i.e. the HbS concentration is approximately 3.5 g/dl
E. **False**

Q14
A. **True**
B. **False** – A recent myocardial infarction (MI) or significant coronary artery disease increases the risk of peri-operative MI
C. **True**
D. **False** – Isoflurane stabilises blood pressure during anaesthesia
E. **False** – There is no association

Q15
A. **True** – A pacemaker is needed regardless of surgery
B. **True** – A pacemaker is needed regardless of surgery
C. **False** – This is no longer an indication for pacemaking
D. **False** – Atrial fibrillation may be treated with digoxin
E. **False**

3. Infection

Q1   Necrotising fasciitis (NF):

A. Results from synergism between aerobic and anaerobic organisms
B. Is more common in immunocompromised patients
C. Of the abdominal wall is called MacEwen's gangrene
D. Requires treatment mainly with high doses of IV antibiotics
E. Is characterised by muscle necrosis

Q2   The AIDS virus (HIV):

A. Binds to CD4 molecules on helper T cells
B. Is more contagious than hepatitis B virus
C. Reverse transcriptase is inhibited by cyclosporin A
D. Has a seroconversion rate of 0.5% following needlestick injuries
E. Infection is usually diagnosed by positive isolation of HIV 1 from the peripheral blood

Q3   The clinical features of AIDS include:

A. Fall in CD8:CD4 ratio in the peripheral blood
B. Hypergammaglobulinaemia
C. Thrombocytopenia
D. Bowel perforation
E. Anal ulceration

Q4   Hepatitis B virus:

A. Contains DNA in its core
B. Has a carrier rate of approximately 0.1% in south-east Asia
C. Antigen presence in serum indicates increased infectivity
D. Surface antigen antibody usually appears within 2 weeks of infection
E. Is a recognised cause of hepatic carcinoma

Q5   The identifying criteria of *Staphylococcus aureus* include:

A. Coagulase positivity
B. Phosphatase negativity
C. Fermentation of mannitol
D. Fluorescent greenish appearance of colonies
E. Serology by identification of Lancefield groups

Q6   *Actinomyces israeli*:

A. Is a true bacterium
B. Is a strict aerobe
C. Causes a chronic granulomatous infection with pus discharge containing yellow-brown sulphur granules
D. Most commonly affects the ileocaecal region in actinomycosis
E. Is usually sensitive to penicillin

Q7   **With respect to some surgically important infections:**

A. Osteomyelitis is a recognised complication of boils
B. Carbuncles are usually caused by *Streptococcus pyogenes*
C. Erysipelas is usually caused by *Erysipelothrix rhusiopathiae*
D. *Clostridium difficile* colitis responds to ciprofloxacin
E. The production of coagulase by *Streptococcus pyogenes* explains its invasiveness in cellulitis

Q8   **The pathophysiological effects of endotoxins include:**

A. Initial leucopenia
B. Release of interleukin 1
C. Inhibition of Hageman factor
D. Activation of the alternative complement pathway
E. Stimulation of platelet aggregation

Q9   **Clostridial gas gangrene:**

A. Is caused by Gram-positive obligate anaerobes
B. Is a recognised cause of progressive haemolytic anaemia
C. May be treated by placing the patient in a pure oxygen chamber at 13 atmospheres for a few hours daily
D. Produces pathological and clinical features that are mainly caused by endotoxins
E. Is relatively common in lower limb amputations for peripheral vascular disease

Q10 *Staphylococcus aureus* **is usually responsible for abscess formation in the following sites:**

A. Appendix
B. Axilla
C. Finger pulp
D. Ischiorectal region
E. Breast

Q11 **The following bacteria may cause gas gangrene:**

A. *Clostridium septicum*
B. *Clostridium histolyticum*
C. *Staphylococcus aureus*
D. *Listeria monocytogenes*
E. *Clostridium novyi* (*oedematiens*)

Q12 *Staphylococcus aureus*:

A. Possesses leucocidins
B. Is resistant to phagocytosis by polymorphonuclear leucocytes
C. Is usually responsible for carbuncles
D. Phage type III is the commonest cause of boils
E. Is usually sensitive to fusidic acid

Q13 The following antimicrobials act by inhibiting the cell wall synthesis of the microbe:

A. Cefuroxime
B. Vancomycin
C. Erythromycin
D. Gentamicin
E. Amphotericin B

Answers to Section 3

Q1
A. **True**
B. **True**
C. **False** – It is called Meleney's gangrene. NF of the scrotum is called Fournier's gangrene
D. **False** – Urgent surgical excision combined with IV antibiotics is the mainstay of treatment
E. **False** – Necrosis of the subcutaneous tissue and fascia is characteristic

Q2
A. **True**
B. **False** – It is less contagious
C. **False** – Cyclosporin A is an immunosuppressant drug. AZT can inhibit the virus reverse transcriptase
D. **True**
E. **False** – The diagnosis is usually made by demonstrating viral antibodies by ELISA or immunoblotting

Q3
A. **False** – The CD8:CD4 ratio rises, the CD4:CD8 ratio falls
B. **True** – Due to polyclonal activation of B lymphocytes
C. **True**
D. **True** – Due to cytomegalovirus (CMV) infection
E. **True** – Due to lymphoma, Kaposi's sarcoma, squamous cell carcinoma, CMV or cryptosporidium

Q4
A. **True**
B. **False** – This is true of the UK. The carrier rate reaches 10–15% in parts of Africa and south-east Asia
C. **True** – The presence of DNA polymerase also indicates increased infectivity
D. **False** – HBsAb appears late and indicates immunity
E. **True**

Q5
A. **True**
B. **False** – It is phosphatase positive
C. **True**
D. **False** – The colonies are typically golden but pigmentation ranges from orange to white
E. **False** – This applies to *Streptococcus*

Q6
A. **True**
B. **False** – It is a strict anaerobe
C. **True**
D. **False** – The ileocaecal region is involved in about 20% of cases. Cervicofacial actinomycosis is the commonest, accounting for about 65% of cases
E. **True**

Q7
A. **True**
B. **False** – They are caused by *Staphylococcus aureus*
C. **False** – It is usually caused by *Streptococcus*
D. **False** – Oral vancomycin or metronidazole is the recognised treatment
E. **False** – The production of hyaluronidase and streptokinase explains the invasiveness

Q8
A. **True**
B. **True** – Causing fever
C. **False**
D. **True**
E. **True**

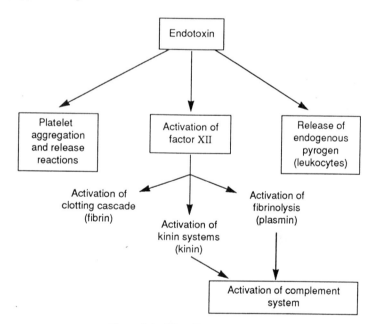

Figure 3.1   The effects of endotoxin

Q9
A. **True**
B. **True** – Due to exotoxins
C. **False** – The patient is placed in pure oxygen at 3 atmospheres
D. **False** – They are caused by exotoxins
E. **True** – Due to local hypoxia

Q10

A. **False** – Faecal flora and *Streptococcus milleri* are usually responsible here
B. **True**
C. **True** – Through a penetrating wound
D. **False** – Faecal flora from the rectum including *E. coli* and anaerobes are usually responsible here
E. **True**

Q11

A. **True**
B. **True**
C. **False**
D. **False**
E. **True**

Q12

A. **True**
B. **False** – It is readily phagocytosed by these cells but the polymorphs are killed after phagocytosis
C. **True**
D. **False** – The main cause is *Staphylococcus aureus* phage type I and II
E. **True**

Q13

A. **True**
B. **True**
C. **False** – It inhibits protein synthesis in ribosomes
D. **False** – It inhibits protein synthesis in ribosomes
E. **False** – It interferes with the barrier function of the cell membrane

4. Anaesthesia and Intensive Care

Q1   In adult respiratory distress syndrome (ARDS):

A. Computed tomography (CT) is a useless investigation
B. The functional residual capacity of the lung is usually reduced
C. There is depletion of type I pneumocytes
D. There is significant improvement in symptoms with the use of frusemide
E. Mechanical ventilation is usually indicated if $PaO_2 < 8\,kPa$

Q2   The clinical features of adult respiratory distress syndrome (not complicated by cardiac failure) include:

A. Increased pulmonary capillary wedge pressure (PCWP)
B. Widespread bilateral infiltrate on chest radiography
C. Increased lung compliance
D. Increased right to left shunting
E. Tachycardia

Q3   Propofol:

A. Causes pain on intravenous injection
B. At a dose of 2.5 mg/kg produces chemical hypnosis which lasts for 25 minutes
C. Has been reported to cause convulsions
D. Should not be used with antimuscarinic drugs
E. Is used to sedate patients in intensive care units

Q4   Suxamethonium:

A. Is a non-depolarising muscle relaxant
B. Causes fasciculations
C. Induces muscular paralysis that lasts for 45 minutes
D. Is contraindicated in liver failure
E. Action can be reversed

Q5   The cardiorespiratory effects of the pneumoperitoneum in laparoscopic surgery include:

A. Increased lung volumes
B. Increased airway resistance
C. Decreased venous return
D. Increased intrathoracic pressure
E. Increased pulmonary compliance

Q6   Lignocaine:

A. 1% solution contains 100 mg/ml
B. Efficacy as a local anaesthetic is increased in the presence of a low pH
C. Maximum safe dose almost doubles when adrenaline is added
D. May cause ventricular dysrhythmias
E. Maximum safe dose for a 70 kg adult is approximately 200 mg (no adrenaline)

Q7   Controlled ventilation results in:

A. A positive peak of intrapleural pressure at the end of expiration
B. An increase in vena cava blood flow during inspiration
C. An increase in lobar pulmonary blood flow during inspiration
D. An apparent rise in central venous pressure
E. An increase in cardiac output

Q8   The consequences of spinal anaesthesia include:

A. Hypotension
B. Relaxation of bowel muscles
C. Headaches
D. Reduction of the three-month mortality rate in patients with hip fractures undergoing surgery
E. Increased muscle tone

Q9   The following drugs are suitable sedatives for use in intensive care:

A. Propofol
B. Morphine
C. Etomidate
D. Midazolam
E. Neostigmine

Q10   During cardiopulmonary resuscitation:

A. A precordial 'thump' is the first line of treatment after basic resuscitation
B. 1 µg of adrenaline is recommended for electromechanical dissociation in an adult
C. Atropine is recommended for asystole
D. The initial DC shock in an adult is 200 J
E. Atropine is recommended for electromechanical dissociation

Q11   Recognised complications of epidural infusions of bupivacaine plus opioid for postoperative pain include:

A. Hypertension
B. Itching
C. Urinary retension
D. Hyperventilation
E. Sedation

Q12   Pulse oximetry:

A. Is based on Beer's law
B. Usually uses four wavelengths of light
C. Readings of 95% correspond approximately to a PCO_2 of 16 kPa
D. Using an ear probe is less rapid but more precise than that using a finger probe
E. Tends to underestimate oxygen saturation in the presence of nail polish

Q13 Pulse oximeters:

A. Have a mean error of < 2%
B. Give readings that are not influenced by methaemoglobinaemia
C. Give readings of oxygen saturation instantaneously
D. May be influenced by surgical diathermy
E. Tend to show a large over-estimation, the lower the saturation of arterial oxygen

Q14 The following monitoring equipment should be available to the anaesthetist during anaesthesia:

A. Capnograph
B. Pulse oximeter
C. Disconnection alarm
D. Peripheral nerve stimulator
E. Oxygen analyser

Q15 Tracheostomy for mechanical ventilation (rather than endotracheal intubation):

A. Improves tracheal toilet
B. Allows earlier enteral feeding
C. Increases sedation requirements
D. Increases the incidence of nosocomial pneumonia
E. Increases the work of breathing

Q16 Frusemide:

A. Is extensively bound to albumin
B. Increases renal blood flow
C. Improves left ventricular ejection fraction
D. Has a similar effect on potassium excretion to that of captopril
E. Reduces urinary calcium excretion

Q17 Septic shock:

A. Is usually caused by Gram-positive bacteria
B. Is characterised by compensatory vasoconstriction
C. Causes myocardial depression
D. Is associated with hepatic failure
E. Is commonly treated with dopamine and noradrenaline

Q18 Atracurium:

A. Is a non-depolarising muscle relaxant
B. Has a half-life of 20 minutes
C. Action is potentiated by halothane
D. Is contraindicated in liver disease
E. Has significant autonomic side effects

Q19 Halothane:

A. Is flammable
B. Inhalation induction is inferior to that of isoflurane
C. Induces hepatitis with an incidence of 1:150 000
D. Induction of hepatitis may be genetically determined
E. Increases renal plasma flow

Q20 Non-steroidal anti-inflammatory drugs (NSAIDs):

A. Inhibit cyclooxygenase
B. May cause respiratory depression
C. Potentiate warfarin effects
D. Are a recognised cause of acute interstitial nephritis
E. Are not hepatotoxic

Q21 Midazolam:

A. Is water insoluble
B. Is shorter acting than diazepam
C. Is well absorbed from mucosal surfaces
D. Given i.m. is less effective than opiates as a premedication
E. Has a predictable first-pass metabolism

Q22 The following drugs may be used to reverse general anaesthesia

A. Neostigmine
B. Mivacurium
C. Naloxone
D. Atropine
E. Phenoxybenzamine

Q23 Nitrous oxide:

A. Is satisfactory as a sole anaesthetic
B. Is used in a concentration of 50–70% with oxygen in anaesthesia
C. Administration is safe in the presence of pneumothorax
D. Has analgesic properties
E. May cause megaloblastic anaemia

Q24 Recognised contraindications to the use of suxamethonium in anaesthesia include:

A. Plasma pseudocholinesterase deficiency
B. Family history of malignant hyperpyrexia
C. Epilepsy
D. Rheumatoid arthritis
E. Diabetes mellitus

Q25   The complications of total parenteral nutrition (TPN) include:

A. Hyperosmolar diuresis
B. Air embolism
C. Septicaemia
D. Liver failure
E. Thrombophlebitis migrans

Q26   With central venous catheters:

A. The subclavian access is less hazardous than the internal jugular vein access
B. The patient should be tilted in the head-up position during the insertion
C. It is advisable to use an electrocardiograph monitor during catheterisation
D. The catheter is usually radiolucent
E. The normal catheter venous pressure is 2–10 cm of saline

Q27   The effects of positive pressure ventilation (PPV) used in anaesthesia include:

A. Decreased cardiac output
B. Increased pulmonary vascular resistance
C. Decreased functional residual capacity
D. Increased antidiuretic hormone (ADH) and aldosterone secretion
E. Decreased intracranial pressure if the patient is hyperventilated

Q28   The consequences of acute upper airway obstruction include:

A. Cyanosis
B. Bradycardia
C. A rise in blood pH
D. Polycythaemia
E. Inspiratory stridor

Q29   The haemoglobin–oxygen dissociation curve is shifted to the right in:

A. Pyrexia
B. Respiratory acidosis
C. States of decreased concentration of 2,3-diphosphoglycerate inside the red cell
D. Polycythaemia
E. Sickle cell anaemia

Q30   Nociception (pain):

A. Is transmitted faster through C fibres than through A fibres
B. Ascends through the spinothalamic tract
C. Of autonomic nature is usually well localised
D. Transmission is facilitated by the stimulation of μ receptors in the central nervous system
E. In disseminated cancer may be relieved by hypophysectomy

Q31 Femoral nerve block:

A. Permits femoral hernia repair
B. Reduces the pain of femoral neck fractures
C. Is contraindicated in patients with peripheral vascular disease (PVD)
D. Is administered by injection medial to the femoral artery
E. Permits surgical excision of the patella

Q32 Morphine:

A. Undergoes negligible first-pass metabolism when given orally
B. Is mainly eliminated unchanged by the kidneys
C. Produces a useful analgesia that lasts approximately 5 hours
D. Stimulates the chemoreceptor trigger zone
E. May be beneficial in a patient with left ventricular failure

Q33 Lignocaine when used as a local anaesthetic:

A. Inhibits the rapid inflow of Na^+ into excitable cells
B. Reduces the resting transmembrane potential of excitable cells
C. Is more active if injected into an inflamed area
D. May cause cardiac arrest
E. Has a local anaesthetic action lasting for about 1 hour (1% lignocaine)

Answers to Section 4

Q1
A. **False** – CT may allow quantification of lung damage
B. **True**
C. **True** – Interstitial haemorrhage, oedema and leucocyte infiltration of alveoli are typical findings
D. **False** – However, cardiac failure may complicate the syndrome in the later stages
E. **True** – Intermittent positive pressure or positive end expiratory pressure ventilation may be used

Q2
A. **False** – The pulmonary capillary wedge pressure (PCWP) is usually normal. It is increased in left ventricular failure
B. **True** – This is characteristic
C. **False** – Lung compliance is reduced
D. **True**
E. **True** – Dyspnoea, tachycardia and tachypnoea are the usual symptoms

Q3
A. **True** – Therefore it should not be injected into a small vein; addition of local anaesthetic such as lignocaine may be useful
B. **False** – It lasts for 5 minutes
C. **True**
D. **False** – Propofol may cause bradycardia, and antimuscarinics may be added to prevent this
E. **True**

Q4
A. **False** – It is a depolarising relaxant
B. **True**
C. **False** – Its action lasts for approximately 5 minutes
D. **True** – It is also contraindicated in burns, pseudocholinesterase deficiency and where there is a family history of malignant hyperpyrexia
E. **False** – Its action cannot be reversed (unlike that of non-depolarising relaxants)

Q5
A. **False** – Lung volumes decrease
B. **True**
C. **True**
D. **True**
E. **False** – Pulmonary compliance is reduced

Q6
A. **False** – 1% solution contains 10 mg/ml
B. **False** – Acidosis reduces its efficacy
C. **True**
D. **True**
E. **True** – 3 mg/kg without adrenaline. When adrenaline is added, the maximum safe dose becomes 500 mg in such a patient

Q7
A. **False** – The positive peak occurs during inspiration
B. **False** – The thoracic pump mechanism is abolished during controlled ventilation, thus reducing venous return and cardiac output
C. **False** – The reduced cardiac putput and increased intrathoracic pressure lead to decreased pulmonary blood flow
D. **True** – This may reflect the rise in intrathoracic pressure
E. **False**

Q8
A. **True** – Due to decreased peripheral resistance
B. **False** – The bowel contracts owing to loss of sympathetic innervation
C. **True** – Due to CSF leakage
D. **False**
E. **False** – There is profound muscular relaxation

Q9
A. **True**
B. **True**
C. **False** – Etomidate is a recognised cause of adrenocortical suppression
D. **True**
E. **False** – This drug inhibits cholinesterase, thus enhancing cholinergic activity

Q10
A. **True**
B. **False** – 1 mg (1 ml of 1:1000) adrenaline is recommended
C. **True**
D. **True**
E. **False** – Adrenaline is recommended for asystole

Q11
A. **False** – Hypotension commonly ensues
B. **True**
C. **True**
D. **False** – Hypoventilation is a recognised complication
E. **True**

Q12

A. **True** – Beer's law indicates that the concentration of a solute can be determined by light absorption
B. **False** – Two wavelengths are usually used
C. **False** – Corresponds to about 10 kPa
D. **False** – Finger probes are less rapid but more precise
E. **True**

Q13

A. **True**
B. **False** – Methaemoglobinaemia tends to reduce readings to about 85%
C. **False** – They take 3–10 s
D. **True**
E. **True**

Q14

A. **True**
B. **True**
C. **True**
D. **True**
E. **True**

Q15

A. **True**
B. **True**
C. **False** – Sedation requirements are reduced
D. **False** – The incidence is reduced
E. **False** – The work of breathing is reduced

Q16

A. **True**
B. **True** – By decreasing renal vascular resistance
C. **True**
D. **False** – Frusemide causes hypokalaemia; captopril decreases potassium excretion by the kidney
E. **False** – It increases calcium excretion
Note: It is important to ensure adequate vascular volume prior to the use of frusemide

Q17

A. **False** – Gram-negative bacteria are usually responsible
B. **False** – Peripheral vasodilatation occurs as a result of mediators triggered by the endotoxin
C. **True**
D. **True**
E. **True**

Q18
A. **True** – Therefore its action is reversible
B. **True**
C. **True** – Enflurane has the least potentiating effect
D. **False** – Its excretion is not influenced by liver failure
E. **False** – It is relatively free of autonomic side effects

Q19
A. **False**
B. **True**
C. **False** – The incidence is about 1:35000
D. **True**
E. **False** – It reduces renal blood flow, probably by increasing renal vascular resistance

Q20
A. **True** – Thus reducing prostaglandin synthesis
B. **False** – This is a side effect of opiates
C. **True** – By displacing warfarin from albumin and acting as antiplatelets
D. **True**
E. **False** – Hepatotoxicity may occur with all NSAIDs

Q21
A. **False** – It is water soluble
B. **True**
C. **True** – Therefore it can be given rectally, sublingually or intravenously
D. **False** – It is more effective
E. **False** – Despite this, it is effective orally

Q22
A. **True** – Cholinesterase inhibitors may be used to reverse muscle relaxants
B. **False** – This is a non-depolarising muscle relaxant
C. **True** – To reverse narcotics
D. **True** – May be given before a cholinesterase inhibitor to reduce cholinergic side effects
E. **False** – This is an α-blocker mainly used in phaeochromocytoma

Q23
A. **False**
B. **True**
C. **False** – Nitrous oxide may diffuse into the pneumothorax, causing enlargement, and may compromise respiration
D. **True** – Entonox contains 50% nitrous oxide and 50% oxygen
E. **True** – After prolonged exposure, due to interference with vitamin B12 action

Q24
A. **True** – Suxamethonium is metabolised by plasma pseudocholinesterase
B. **True** – Suxamethonium is a recognised trigger of this potentially fatal condition
C. **False**
D. **False**
E. **False**

Q25
A. **True**
B. **True** – Other catheter complications include pneumothorax, haemothorax, thrombosis, haemorrhage and cardiac dysrhythmias
C. **True**
D. **True**
E. **False** – This is a recognised feature of pancreatic cancer

Q26
A. **False** – The subclavian access is more hazardous
B. **False** – The patient should be tilted in the head-down position to distend the vein and reduce the risk of embolism
C. **True** – When the catheter passes beyond the right atrium, cardiac dysrhythmias may ensue
D. **False** – Radio-opaque catheters detectable on radiography are used
E. **True**

Q27
A. **True** – Due to decreased venous return, depressed ventricular performance and increased pulmonary vascular resistance
B. **True**
C. **False** – This increases by about 17%
D. **True** – Due to decreased renal perfusion
E. **True**

Q28
A. **True**
B. **True** – This is a dangerous sign
C. **False** – There is respiratory acidosis (increased PCO_2 lowers pH)
D. **False**
E. **True**

Q29
A. **True**
B. **True**
C. **False** – This shifts the curve to the left
D. **False** – This shifts the curve to the left
E. **True**

Q30
A. **False** – It is faster through the myelinated A fibres
B. **True**
C. **False** – Autonomic pain is ill defined and felt as a dull ache, whereas somatic pain is sharp and localised
D. **False** – Stimulation of μ receptors (usually by opiates) produces analgesia
E. **True**

Q31

A. **False** – The femoral hernia region is not part of the blocked field
B. **True**
C. **False** – Femoral block is recommended in patients with PVD, but solutions containing vasoconstrictors should be avoided
D. **False** –The femoral nerve is located lateral to the artery
E. **False** – Femoral nerve block is inadequate for operations on the patella

Q32

A. **False** – Extensive first-pass metabolism occurs
B. **False** – Morphine undergoes both hepatic and renal metabolism and only 10% of the drug is excreted unchanged in urine
C. **True** – $t_{1/2}$ is 2–4 hours
D. **True** – Causing nausea and vomiting
E. **True** – Venodilatation relieves the pre-load of the heart

Q33

A. **True** – By displacing Ca^{2+} from its sites on membrane phospholipids
B. **False** – The resting potential is unaffected
C. **False** – Lignocaine is a weak base ($ROH \rightleftharpoons R^+ + OH^-$). The local tissue acidosis, due to inflammation, shifts the dissociation reaction to the right so that more of the drug is in the lipid-insoluble form (ionised)
D. **True** – This is a recognised adverse effect
E. **True**

5. The Operating Theatre/Sutures

Q1   Diathermy:

A. Means "coagulation"
B. Uses an electrosurgical unit that converts 50 Hz AC into 50 000 Hz AC
C. Current follows the pathway of maximal resistance
D. Causes less surrounding tissue damage when used in the monopolar form (than in the bipolar form)
E. Of the monopolar type is used in circumcision

Q2   Catgut sutures:

A. Consist of twisted collagen derived from the intestines of sheep
B. Are absorbed by phagocytes
C. Are stronger than polydioxanone (PDS®) suture
D. Handle and tie better than polyglactin (Vicryl®) sutures
E. Are useful in intestinal anastomosis

Q3   Autoclaving:

A. Is the most frequently used method of sterilisation
B. Kills the spores of *Clostridium botulinum*
C. Utilises dry heat at 180°C
D. Is primarily used for glassware sterilisation
E. Requires 15–20 minutes for sterilisation

Q4   The following techniques are used to reduce exogenous bacterial contamination of the air in theatres:

A. Infrared irradiation
B. Laminar air flow
C. Wearing of exhaust ventilated non-porous clothing by theatre staff
D. Ultraviolet irradiation
E. Wearing of masks by theatre staff

Q5   Skin preparation:

A. Iodine (2% in 50% ethanol) can sterilise the patient's skin
B. Shaving should be performed 24 hours before surgery
C. Sterile adhesive plastic skin drapes have been shown to reduce infection rate (compared with traditional drapes)
D. Bathing with chlorhexidine detergent reduces the bacterial burden of the groin and axilla
E. *Staphylococcus epidermidis* is the commonest contaminant

Q6   The following are synthetic non-absorbable sutures:

A. Polypropylene
B. Polyglycolic acid
C. Polyamide
D. Polydioxanone
E. Polyester

Q7   In the operating theatre environment:

A. Humidity should be approximately 10%
B. The ambient temperature is usually 17°C
C. There are 20–40 air changes per hour
D. The use of vertical laminar air flow, exhaust suits and plastic tents has been shown to reduce infection risk in total hip replacement
E. 0.5 parts per 1000 of halothane is an acceptable level of contamination

Q8   In monopolar diathermy:

A. The patient plate should be sited far away from the operating site
B. The plate site should be prepared with antiseptic prior to plate application
C. A cardiac pacemaker is a relative contraindication
D. The patient's body must not touch the metal drip stand
E. Misapplication of the patient plate is the commonest cause of diathermy burns

Q9   In limb surgery:

A. Tourniquets are contraindicated in peripheral vascular disease
B. The tourniquet maximal pressure should be 500 mmHg for the upper limb
C. The maximal duration of tourniquet application is 4 hours for safe use
D. Exsanguinating the limb with an Esmarch bandage is contraindicated in suspected deep vein thrombosis involving the limb
E. Compartment syndrome is a recognised complication of tourniquet use

Q10   During operations on patients infected with HIV:

A. The risk of seroconversion following a needlestick injury is 1:1000
B. The number of staff should be reduced to a minimum
C. Double gloving is recommended
D. It is advisable to cover the operating table with a sheet of polythene
E. Gloves and eye protection are not necessary for endoscopic procedures

Answers to Section 5

Q1
A. **False** – It means "heating through"
B. **True** – This is the basic principle. The hazardous current is converted into a therapeutic current
C. **False** – The less resistant pathway is followed
D. **False** – Bipolar diathermy causes less tissue damage. Only tissue held between the forceps is heated
E. **False** – Monopolar diathermy is contraindicated in circumcision. Catgut sutures are used for haemostasis. Bipolar diathermy can also be used

Q2
A. **True**
B. **True**
C. **False** – They are weaker
D. **False** – Vicryl handles and ties better
E. **True**

Q3
A. **True**
B. **True**
C. **False** – It utilises moist steam at 121°C and a pressure of 15 lb/in^2
D. **False** – Glassware is usually sterilised by dry heat (180°C)
E. **True**

Q4
A. **False**
B. **True** – This has been shown to reduce wound infection in arthroplasty operations
C. **True**
D. **True**
E. **False** – There is no evidence that this reduces exogenous bacterial contamination

Q5
A. **False** – Skin sterilisation (removal of all micro-organisms) is impossible
B. **False** – This results in a higher rate of contamination and infection. Shaving immediately before the operation is to be preferred
C. **False**
D. **True** – The impact of this on wound infection rate is controversial
E. **True**

Q6
A. **True** – This suture is synthetic and non-absorbable (Prolene®)
B. **False** – This suture is synthetic and absorbable (Dexon®)
C. **True** – Commercially known as nylon
D. **False** – This suture is synthetic and absorbable (PDS®)
E. **True** – This is Dacron®

Q7
A. **False** – It should be approximately 50%
B. **False** – 20–24°C is acceptable
C. **True**
D. **True**
E. **False** – 0.5 parts per 10^6 is the maximal acceptable level

Q8
A. **False** – It should be close to the operating site
B. **False** – Skin preparations should not be allowed to seep under the plate
C. **True** – Cardiac dysrhythmias may ensue: monothermal diathermy should be avoided in the presence of a pacemaker, but polar diathermy can be used
D. **True** – Earthed metal objects may cause diathermy burns
E. **True**

Q9
A. **True**
B. **False** – 250 mmHg is the maximal pressure for the upper limb and 500 mmHg for the lower limb
C. **False** – Maximal duration is 2 hours
D. **True** – Infection is another contraindication
E. **True** – Due to ischaemia

Q10
A. **False** – The risk is approximately 0.5%
B. **True**
C. **True**
D. **True**
E. **False** – Gloves and eye protection should be worn

6. Skin and Wounds

Q1 The following types of operation and risks of clinical wound infection are correctly paired:

A. Clean – 3%
B. Hartmann's procedure for colonic perforation – 10%
C. Inguinal herniorrhaphy – 10%
D. Clean contaminated – 12%
E. Cholecystectomy – 3%

Q2 The following are suitable recipient sites for split-thickness skin grafts:

A. Cartilage denuded of perichondrium
B. Exposed muscle tendons
C. A thigh wound containing 10^5 B-haemolytic streptococci per gram of tissue
D. Bone denuded of periosteum
E. A non-infected venous leg ulcer 7 cm in diameter

Q3 Keloid scars:

A. Invade nearby normal tissue
B. May be treated with topical triamcinolone
C. Have an increased incidence after postoperative radiotherapy
D. Commonly cause pruritus
E. Contain less collagen than "normal" scars

Q4 The following factors increase the incidence of wound dehiscence:

A. Corticosteroid therapy
B. Chronic obstructive airways disease
C. Previous radiotherapy
D. Malnutrition
E. Overtightened sutures

Q5 Split-thickness skin grafts:

A. Contain a portion of the dermis
B. Can survive on bone denuded of periosteum
C. Develop a true circulation within 1 week
D. Are cosmetically superior to full-thickness grafts
E. Can be stored for later use

Q6 Compared with split-thickness (ST) grafts, full-thickness (FT) skin grafts have:

A. A larger supply of donor sites
B. Less secondary contracture
C. A higher "take" rate
D. Greater durability
E. An inferior cosmetic outcome

Q7 Random flaps:

A. Have an anatomically recognised arterial and venous system
B. May be transferred as free flaps and transplanted to other sites
C. Have a more reliable blood supply than axial flaps
D. Include Z-plasty
E. Include V–Y advancement flap

Q8 The incidence of wound infection can be reduced by the use of:

A. Starch-free gloves rather than starch-coated gloves
B. Mechanical bowel preparation in colorectal surgery
C. Laminar air flow in theatres
D. Intravenous antibiotics in joint replacement operations
E. Braided non-absorbable sutures (rather than monofilamentous non-absorbable sutures)

Q9 The following myocutaneous flaps (MFs) and vascular pedicles are correctly paired:

A. Latissimus dorsi MF – subscapular artery
B. Transverse rectus abdominis MF – superficial circumflex iliac artery
C. Tensor fascia lata MF – transverse branch of the lateral femoral circumflex artery
D. Gracilis MF – lateral femoral circumflex artery
E. Pectoralis major MF – thoracoacromial artery

Q10 In a small wound healing by first intention which has been sutured by mono-filamentous nylon (assuming no complications):

A. Monocytes help to clean away the debris by phagocytosis
B. The epidermal and dermal epithelia grow downwards along the suture track
C. Fibroblasts have a contractile function which helps to produce a small scar
D. Early removal of sutures does not influence the extent of the granulomatous response
E. The wound site is as vascular during the fourth week as during the first week of healing

Q11 When a clean incision is sutured with the skin edges being closely apposed (assuming no complications):

A. The process of healing is referred to as healing by second intention
B. There is usually no acute inflammatory reaction associated with the process of healing
C. New collagen is demonstrable in the wound by the second day
D. Reticulin is demonstrable in the wound by the third day
E. A continuous layer of epidermis usually forms in 48 hours

Q12 The following factors impair wound healing:

A. Zinc deficiency
B. Previous radiotherapy
C. Uraemia
D. Rheumatoid arthritis
E. Ultraviolet light

Q13 The following favour a good prognosis in melanoma:

A. Male sex
B. A low Breslow's thickness
C. Older age
D. Hutchinson's freckle type
E. A high Clark's level

Q14 Squamous cell carcinoma is a recognised complication of:

A. Actinic keratosis
B. Squamous cell papilloma
C. Basal cell papilloma
D. Bowen's disease
E. Compound naevus

Q15 Basal cell carcinoma:

A. Spread to regional lymph nodes has been reported
B. Ulcer is characterised by an everted edge
C. Over the nasal cartilage is best treated with radiotherapy
D. Frequently arises from basal cell papilloma
E. Usually arises in the mask area of the face

Q16 Pilonidal sinus:

A. Is usually congenital
B. Is more common in males
C. Literally means "nest of hairs"
D. Recurrence after surgery is not reduced by regular shaving of the adjacent skin
E. Wounds after excision are frequently left open

Answers to Section 6

Q1
A. **True**
B. **False** – This is a contaminated operation associated with a higher infection rate
C. **False** – This is a clean operation and the risk is approximately 3%
D. **True**
E. **False** – This is a clean contaminated operation with a 12% risk of wound infection

Q2
A. **False**
B. **False**
C. **False**
D. **False**
E. **True**

Q3
A. **True**
B. **True** – This potent steroid is injected intradermally
C. **False** – Postoperative radiotherapy is used to decrease incidence (24 hours after operation)
D. **True**
E. **False** – Keloid scars contain higher levels of collagen and fibroblast activity

Q4
A. **True**
B. **True** – Due to hypoxia and increased intra-abdominal pressure
C. **True** – Radiotherapy may cause obliteration of small vessels causing local ischaemia
D. **True**
E. **True** – Due to resulting local ischaemia

Q5
A. **True**
B. **False**
C. **True**
D. **False** – They are cosmetically inferior to full-thickness grafts
E. **True** – In normal saline (at 4°C)

Q6
A. **True** – FT grafts have limited donor sites
B. **True**
C. **False** – ST grafts have better take rates
D. **True**
E. **False** – FT grafts are better in this respect

Q7

A. **False** – Such a system is lacking. The blood supply is derived from the dermal–subdermal plexus
B. **False** – This is true of axial and myocutaneous flaps
C. **False** – They have a less reliable blood supply
D. **True**
E. **True**

Q8

A. **False** – Starch has been shown to increase the incidence of intra-abdominal adhesions
B. **True** – e.g. magnesium sulphate
C. **True**
D. **True** – Prophylactic antibiotics should be given at induction of anaesthesia
E. **False** – The infection risk is less with monofilamentous sutures

Q9

A. **False** – Thoracodorsal artery
B. **False** – Inferior and superior epigastric arteries
C. **True**
D. **False** – Medial femoral circumflex artery
E. **True**

Q10

A. **True**
B. **True** – To form an incomplete tube of epithelium around the suture
C. **True**
D. **False** – Early removal decreases the extent of granulation
E. **False** – The vascular elements decrease with time until the scar becomes almost avascular

Q11

A. **False** – It is healing by first intention
B. **False** – A mild acute inflammatory reaction usually occurs within 24 hours
C. **False** – It is demonstrable by the fifth day
D. **True**
E. **True**

Q12

A. **True**
B. **True** – Due to impaired blood supply
C. **True**
D. **True**
E. **False** – This has been shown to be beneficial to wound healing

Q13

A. **False** – It has a better prognosis in females
B. **True** – The greater the thickness, the worse the prognosis
C. **False** – This is a poor prognostic sign
D. **True** – This is the least aggressive type
E. **True** – However, the concept of melanoma thickness has replaced Clark's level

Q14
A. **True**
B. **False** – This is frequently viral in origin
C. **False** – Also known as seborrhoeic warts
D. **True** – This represents *in situ* carcinoma
E. **False**

Q15
A. **True** – This is rare
B. **False** – The edge is usually rolled
C. **False** – Radiotherapy may cause cartillage collapse due to necrosis. Adequate surgical excision is the mainstay of management
D. **False** – This skin lesion is not pre-malignant
E. **True** – Solar radiation is an important aetiological factor

Q16
A. **False** – It is usually acquired. The congenital form may be associated with dermoid cysts or vestigial glands
B. **True** – It is more common in men who are hairy and aged 20–40 years
C. **True**
D. **False** – Regular shaving reduces recurrence
E. **True** – To heal by secondary intention

7. Fluid and Electrolyte Balance

Q1 Hartmann's solution contains:

A. Albumin
B. 131 mmol of Na^+ (per litre)
C. 10 mmol of K^+ (per litre)
D. No calcium
E. Bicarbonate and lactate

Q2 One litre of 0.9% NaCl and 0.15% of KCl contains:

A. 100 mmol of Na^+
B. 1000 ml of water
C. 300 calories
D. 20 mmol of K^+
E. 150 mmol of Cl^-

Q3 Human albumin solution:

A. Containing 4.5% protein is isotonic
B. Contains clotting factors
C. Is pasteurised
D. Is better retained in the circulation than Haemaccel®
E. Is cheaper than Haemaccel

Q4 Haemaccel:

A. Contains hydroxyethyl starch, which is the osmotically active constituent
B. Can be stored at room temperature
C. Contains 145 mmol of Na^+ per litre
D. Has a longer half-life than starch polymers
E. Does not carry oxygen

Q5 In a healthy 70 kg man living in a temperate climate:

A. The 24 hour urine output is approximately 1400 ml
B. The average insensible water loss is 300 ml per 24 hours
C. 60% of the weight is due to water
D. The 24 hour total sodium loss is 50 mmol
E. The potassium requirement is 60 mmol per day

Q6 The causes of hypocalcaemia include:

A. Thyroidectomy
B. Acute pancreatitis
C. Milk-alkali syndrome
D. Sarcoidosis
E. Magnesium deficiency

Q7   The following are recognised causes of hypercalcaemia:

A. Addison's disease
B. Hypothyroidism
C. Thiazides
D. Long-term immobility
E. Parathyroid carcinoma

Q8   The following are recognised causes of hyponatraemia:

A. Diabetes insipidus
B. Hypothyroidism
C. Adrenocortical deficiency
D. Alcohol
E. Lithium

Q9   The following are recognised causes of hypokalaemia:

A. Frusemide therapy
B. Addison's disease (not associated with hypovolaemic shock)
C. Villous adenoma of the rectum
D. Ileostomy
E. Untreated diabetic ketoacidosis (DKA)

Q10 The following results are compatible with a diagnosis of acute pre-renal failure:

A. A urine sodium concentration of 50 mmol/l
B. A ratio of urine to serum urea concentration of 2.1
C. Serum potassium of 6.0 mmol/l
D. Blood pressure of 85/50
E. Blood pH of 7.30

Q11 Common consequences of chronic renal failure include:

A. Metabolic acidosis
B. Hypercalcaemia
C. Normochromic normocytic anaemia
D. Hypophosphataemia
E. Decreased insulin requirements in an insulin-dependent diabetic patient

Answers to Section 7

Q1
A. **False**
B. **True**
C. **False** – It contains 5 mmol of K^+ (per litre)
D. **False** – It contains 2 mmol of Ca^{2+} per litre
E. **True**

Q2
A. **False** – It contains 150 mmol of Na^+
B. **True**
C. **False** – It contains no calories
D. **True**
E. **True**

Q3
A. **True** – A more concentrated form is also available (15–25%)
B. **False**
C. **True** – To reduce risk of infection
D. **True** – It is particularly valuable in pancreatitis, burns and trauma
E. **False** – It is more expensive

Q4
A. **False** – The active constituent is polygeline (degraded and modified gelatin)
B. **True**
C. **True**
D. **False** – Starch polymers' half-life is longer (6–9 hours). They are also less allergenic
E. **True**

Q5
A. **True**
B. **False** – It is approximately 700 ml
C. **True** – Approximately 43 litres of water
D **False** – It is > 100 mmol of Na^+
E. **True**

Q6
A. **True** – The parathyroid glands may be inadvertently removed
B. **True**
C. **False** – This is an uncommon cause of hypercalcaemia
D. **False** – There is 1-hydroxylation of 25-hydroxycholecalciferol by the macrophages, causing hypercalcaemia
E. **True**

Q7
A. **True**
B. **False** – Thyrotoxicosis may cause hypercalcaemia
C. **True** – Thiazides reduce urinary calcium
D. **True** – Because of bone demineralization
E. **True** – Parathyroid carcinoma is rare. It accounts for 2% of cases of primary hyperparathyroidism

Q8
A. **False** – Diabetes insipidus due to ADH deficiency may cause hypernatraemia
B. **True**
C. **True**
D. **True** – Alcohol stimulates ADH release
E. **False** – Lithium may cause ADH insensitivity and nephrogenic diabetes insipidus (hypernatraemia)

Q9
A. **True** – Frusemide and thiazides increase renal excretion of potassium
B. **False** – Lack of mineralocorticoid activity causes hyperkalaemia
C. **True** – Because of increased gastrointestinal loss of potassium
D. **True** – Because of increased gastrointestinal loss of potassium
E. **False** – Untreated DKA is usually associated with hyperkalaemia. Insulin therapy causes potassium to enter cells and may lead to hypokalaemia

Q10
A. **False** – In pre-renal failure the sodium concentration in urine is usually less than 20 mmol/l due to increased secretion of aldosterone
B. **False** – The ratio of urinary urea to plasma urea is usually > 10
C. **True** – This is due to decreased delivery of Na^+ to the distal tubule
D. **True** – Circulatory insufficiency is the usual cause of acute pre-renal failure
E. **True** – A metabolic acidosis ensues as the excretion of H^+ is reduced (see A)

Q11
A. **True**
B. **False** – Hypocalcaemia usually ensues
C. **True** – This is caused by depression of bone marrow by toxins and by decreased erythropoietin synthesis by the unhealthy kidney
D. **False** – Hyperphosphataemia ensues
E. **True** – This is because insulin is metabolised in the kidneys

8. Blood

Q1 Stored crossmatched blood:

A. pH gradually rises
B. Potassium concentration gradually increases
C. Rapidly loses clotting factors
D. May cause hypothermia when transfused
E. Commonly causes hypercalcaemia after transfusion

Q2 The complications of massive blood transfusion include:

A. Air embolism
B. Hyperkalaemia
C. Thrombocythaemia
D. Disseminated intravascular coagulopathy (DIC)
E. Metabolic alkalosis

Q3 Prolonged thrombin time is usually seen in:

A. Heparin therapy
B. Disseminated intravascular coagulopathy
C. Haemophilia A
D. Warfarin therapy
E. Von Willebrand's disease

Q4 Prothrombin time is increased in:

A. Haemophilia A
B. Von Willebrand's disease
C. Warfarin therapy
D. Heparin therapy
E. Disseminated intravascular coagulopathy

Q5 Causes of thrombocytopenia include:

A. Heparin therapy
B. Haemolytic uraemic syndrome
C. Disseminated intravascular coagulopathy
D. Splenectomy (assuming no significant blood loss)
E. Sarcoidosis

Q6 In haemophilia A:

A. The factor VIII WF Ag level is reduced
B. A factor VIII C level of 20% is adequate for major surgery
C. Desmopressin can elevate factor VIII levels three-fold
D. The half-life of injected factor VIII is 24 hours
E. The inheritance is X-linked recessive

Q7   Causes of disseminated intravascular coagulopathy (DIC) include:

A. Gram-negative septicaemia
B. Hypovolaemia
C. Acute pancreatitis
D. Severe trauma
E. Anaphylactic shock

Q8   In crossmatching of blood for transfusion:

A. The patient's serum is screened for atypical IgM antibodies at 37°C using saline techniques
B. A direct Coombs' test is performed to detect the patient's antibodies to donor red blood cells
C. The erythrocytes from each donor unit are tested against the patient's serum at 37°C to detect IgG antibodies
D. The tests usually take about 1 hour
E. If no time is available, group O rhesus positive blood should be transfused

Q9   In Hodgkin's disease:

A. Lymphocyte-predominant histology is associated with the best prognosis
B. The inguinal region is the commonest site for superficial lymphadenopathy at presentation
C. The presence of Reed–Sternberg cells is essential to the diagnosis
D. The disease does not involve non-lymphatic tissue
E. Cyclical chemotherapy is the treatment of choice in patients with stage I disease

Q10   The laboratory findings in iron-deficiency anaemia include:

A. Normal ferritin
B. Low serum iron
C. Complete absence of iron from macrophages in bone marrow
D. Low total iron binding capacity (TIBC)
E. Decreased mean corpuscular volume (MCV)

Q11   The laboratory findings in disseminated intravascular coagulopathy include:

A. Prolonged thrombin time
B. Low platelet count
C. Elevated levels of fibrinogen degradation products in serum
D. Elevated fibrinogen levels in serum
E. Reduced factor VIII activity

Q12   Idiopathic thrombocytopenic purpura (ITP):

A. Is associated with an autoantibody in most cases
B. Can be treated with intravenous IgG
C. Has a long-term remission rate of 95% when treated by splenectomy
D. Autoantibodies cannot cross the placenta
E. Responds to corticosteroids

Q13 The bleeding time may be prolonged in the following:

A. Von Willebrand's disease
B. Vitamin K deficiency
C. Haemophilia A
D. Idiopathic thrombocytopenic purpura
E. Liver disease

Q14 In haemophilia A:

A. There is a prolonged prothrombin time (PT)
B. The gene coding for the deficient factor is located on the long arm of the X chromo-some
C. Prenatal diagnosis by DNA analysis is possible
D. The gene coding for the deficient factor has been cloned
E. Low levels of the protein VIIIR:Ag are characteristic

Q15 Regarding blood groups and transfusion of blood products:

A. Patients of group O possess anti-A and anti-B antibodies in their serum
B. The possession of antigen d (rather than antigen D) makes the subject rhesus positive (Rh$^+$)
C. Anti-D antibodies are naturally occurring antibodies
D. Cryoprecipitate contains all coagulation factors
E. HLA antibodies are an important cause of febrile transfusion reactions

Answers to Section 8

Q1
A. **False** – It becomes progressively acidic
B. **True** – Due to damaged cells
C. **True**
D. **True** – It is stored at a low temperature (4°C)
E. **False** – Hypocalcaemia may occur, especially if citrate is used for anticoagulation

Q2
A. **True**
B. **True** – Stored blood is rich in K^+ due to cell damage
C. **False** – Platelet content is low: thrombocytopenia may ensue
D. **True** – This can be corrected by fresh frozen plasma
E. **False** – Acidosis may result. Other complications include hypothermia, hypocalcaemia, septicaemia, allergic reactions, and transmission of viral and protozoal infection

Q3
A. **True**
B. **True**
C. **False** – The thrombin time (TT) is normal
D. **False** – The TT is normal
E. **False** – The TT is normal
Note: Thrombin time is determined by adding thrombin to plasma and measuring the time for clot formation

Q4
A. **False** – The prothrombin time (PT) is normal
B. **False** – The PT is normal
C. **True**
D. **True**
E. **True**

Q5
A. **True**
B. **True**
C. **True**
D. **False** – Thrombocytosis usually ensues
E. **False** – Thrombocytosis usually ensues

Q6
A. **False** – Factor VIIIC is reduced, but factor VIII WF Ag is normal
B. **False** – 20% is adequate for minor bleeds. Major surgery requires a 60% level
C. **True**
D. **False** – It is 12 hours, therefore twice daily administration is recommended in the acute episode
E. **True**

Q7
A. **True**
B. **True**
C. **True**
D. **True**
E. **True**

Q8
A. **False** – The detection of IgM antibodies (cold) is carried out at room temperature
B. **False** – The indirect Coombs' test is used for this purpose
C. **True**
D. **True**
E. **False** – Group O rhesus negative blood should be transfused

Q9
A. **True**
B. **False** – The cervical lymph nodes are most commonly involved at presentation
C. **True**
D. **False** – The involvement of non-lymphatic tissue (e.g. skin, lung, brain) usually occurs late
E. **False** – Radiotherapy is the treatment of choice for stages I and II

Q10
A. **False** – The ferritin is usually reduced
B. **True**
C. **True**
D. **False** – The TIBC rises as the saturation decreases due to iron deficiency
E. **True**

Q11
A. **True**
B. **True**
C. **True**
D. **False** – There is fibrinogen deficiency
E. **True**

Q12
A. **True** – In approximately 70% of cases
B. **True**
C. **False** – The long-term remission rate is approximately 70%
D. **False** – The autoantibody (IgG) can cross the placenta, thus causing neonatal thrombocytopenia
E. **True** – Most patients temporarily respond to corticosteroids (up to 3 mg/kg of prednisone)

Q13
A. **True** – Platelet function is impaired
B. **False**
C. **False**
D. **True**
E. **True** – This may cause platelet dysfunction

Q14
A. **False** – The PT is normal
B. **True** – There is X-linked inheritance
C. **True** – After chorionic villous sampling
D. **True**
E. **False** – The level of VIII:C is low (coagulant activity)

Q15
A. **True**
B. **False** – The possession of the D antigen makes the subject Rh^+
C. **False** – These antibodies nearly always arise after immunisation by transfusion or pregnancy
D. **False** – Cryoprecipitate contains factor VIII and fibrinogen. Fresh frozen plasma (FFP) contains all coagulation factors
E. **True**

9.   Postoperative Complications

Q1   In the diagnosis of deep vein thrombosis (DVT):

A. Doppler ultrasonography has a 90% accuracy for calf vein thrombosis
B. Ascending venography is the most accurate investigation
C. Plethysmography has 99% specificity for ileofemoral DVT
D. The differential diagnosis includes ruptured Baker's cyst
E. Homans' sign is reliable

Q2   Consider the postoperative investigation shown in Figure 9.1. The following statements are true:

A. The investigation demonstrates a thrombosis involving the calf, popliteal and femoral veins
B. Doppler ultrasonography is fairly reliable in detecting this complication
C. Radioactive fibrinogen scan is the most accurate investigation to detect this abnormality
D. Unfractionated heparin is more effective in preventing this complication than low molecular weight heparin (LMWH)
E. This patient may develop a leg ulcer

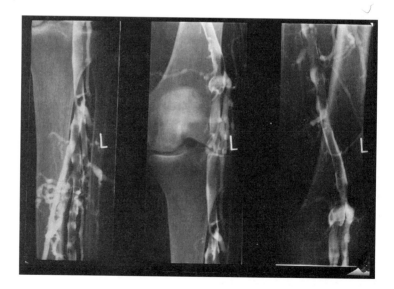

Figure 9.1

7. Regular monitoring of **vital signs**:

- BP

- Pulse respiratory rate

- Temperature

- Urinary output

- Level of consciousness

8. **Find the underlying cause** of shock and plan a definitive treatment. A surgical intervention is often necessary.

Complication	Signs/Symptoms	Prevention	Treatment
Cardiac arrhythmias, myocardial infarction	Tachycardia Hypotension Atrial fibrillation Continuous supraventricular tachycardia Chest pain Shortness of breath Electrocardiographic changes Elevated cardiac enzyme levels	Maintain adequate blood pressure in perioperative period Maintain electrolyte balance Provide adequate pain management Maintain normal body temperature Maintain hemoglobin level at 100 g/L (10 g/dL)or greater[25]	Administer digoxin, diltiazem, β-blockers Use cardioversion Replace electrolytes Use percutaneous transluminal coronary angioplasty Provide oxygen therapy Administer aspirin Administer morphine Administer nitroglycerin
Prolonged ileus	Lack of bowel sounds Increased nasogastric tube drainage Nausea/vomiting No evidence of bowel function for more than 10 days after surgery Decreased appetite	Provide adequate pain management with use of nonnarcotic agents (nonsteroidal anti-inflammatory drugs) Administer metoclopramide Have patient increase activity level	Administer metoclopramide Give stool softeners, suppositories, enemas, bowel stimulants Place a nasogastric tube (by physician) to prevent vomiting
Wound infection	Redness at incision Increased pain at incision Foul odor from wound Swelling at incision Discolored drainage from incision Fever	Administer prophylactic antibiotics Use sterile technique at time of surgery Maintain adequate tissue oxygenation during surgery Maximize nutritional status preoperatively Have staff use meticulous hand washing	Open wound and start dressing changes Administer systemic antibiotics if surrounding erythema significant

Complications	Signs and symptoms	Prevention strategies	Management
Esophageal anastomotic leak	Fever (≥38.6°C [101°F]) Inflammation, pain Drainage from the neck wound or accumulation of fluid at the wound site Subcutaneous emphysema Unexplained tachycardia or tachypnea Hypoxemia Change in color of chest tube drainage[25]	Use skilled surgical techniques Do not feed the patient too early Maintain strict status of no oral intake Manage pain adequately Avoid nasotracheal suctioning after extubation[14]	Use esophagography with water-soluble contrast material to diagnose the leak Increase tube feedings After several days, dilate the esophagus if needed Open neck wound at bedside Irrigate and pack with wet-to-dry dressing Stop oral intake
Pneumonia, adult respiratory distress syndrome, atelectasis	Tachypnea Diminished breath sounds Increased temperature Hypoxemia Poor pulmonary compliance Interstitial infiltrates evident on chest radiograph Dyspnea/shortness of breath Change in mentation Confusion	Have patient stop smoking before surgery Frequently turn patient, and provide use of incentive spirometry, nebulizers Chest physiotherapy, suctioning Feed early after surgery[26] Have patient ambulate early after surgery	Reintubate patient and provide respiratory support as needed Provide appropriate antibiotic therapy Promote aggressive pulmonary toilet Monitor arterial blood gases
Deep vein thrombosis and/or pulmonary emboli	Difficulty breathing Leg swelling Inflammation of involved leg Tachypnea Arrhythmias Pain in leg	Have patient ambulate early after surgery Have patient do leg exercises Provide antiembolism stockings and sequential compression devices Administer subcutaneous heparin	Infuse heparin Maintain bed rest Use a Greenfield filter Provide pulmonary support
Gastric necrosis	Fever	Use skilled surgical techniques	Provide surgery

Management of Hypovolaemic shock – *this needs a rapid treatment

1. Ensure a **patent airway + 100% O2 by mask** or intubation if comatose

2. Patient is placed in **supine** position with elevated legs

3. Establish a **2 large bore IV cannula** access – ideally in the antecubital fossa

   - With shock due to bleeding, take blood for:

     - Cross matching

     - Hb

     - FBC

     - U&E

4. Restore circulating blood volume with **crystalloid initially,** and with plasma expanders or blood as indicated

5. Insert a **central venous line to monitor CVP** and to assess the response to fluid administration

Q3   Anastomotic leak, following an interior resection of the rectum:

A. Usually presents within 24 hours of surgery
B. Is more common if the mesorectum is completely excised
C. Often presents with abdominal pain and pyrexia
D. Should be confirmed by a barium enema
E. Is usually treated surgically by the formation of a colostomy

Q4   Pulmonary embolism:

A. Is associated with deep vein thrombosis (DVT) in approximately 50% of cases
B. Is associated with abnormal plain chest radiography in most cases
C. Is characterised by elevated arterial PCO_2
D. Causes ventilation perfusion mismatch on radioisotope scanning of the lungs
E. Prevention methods include subcutaneous insertion of a filter in the inferior vena cava

Q5   Burst abdomen:

A. Usually declares itself 7–14 days after operation
B. Usually causes severe pain
C. May be caused by over-tightened sutures
D. Incidence is increased in jaundiced patients
E. Is usually treated by immediate reoperation and the use of deep tension sutures

Q6   Postoperative pulmonary collapse:

A. Incidence is not influenced by giving pre-operative breathing exercises
B. Is a common cause of pyrexia 24 hours after operation
C. Is often complicated by infection
D. Is treated mainly using antibiotics
E. May be treated by flexible bronchoscopy

Q7   The following factors increase the risk of postoperative atelectasis

A. Chronic obstructive airways disease
B. Spinal anaesthesia (rather than general anaesthesia)
C. Lower abdominal incisions (rather than upper abdominal incisions)
D. Postoperative epidural analgesia
E. Smoking

Q8   The following are recognised complications of laparoscopic cholecystectomy

A. Tension pneumothorax
B. CO_2 embolism
C. Common bile duct injury
D. Strangulated small bowel obstruction
E. Intraoperative bradycardia

Answers to Section 9

Q1
A. **False** – Doppler ultrasonography is accurate for proximal but not distal DVT
B. **True**
C. **True**
D. **True**
E. **False**

Q2
A. **True** – There is extensive deep vein thrombosis
B. **True** – Venography is the most accurate investigation
C. **False** – This test is time consuming and less accurate than venography
D. **False** – LMWH is more effective and less hazardous
E. **True** – Due to venous hypertension

Q3

A. **False** – It usually presents 5–7 days after operation when the bowel function returns
B. **True** – A defunctioning loop ileostomy may be performed for very low anterior resections
C. **True**
D. **False** – Barium is not water soluble. Water-soluble contrast studies can be useful to confirm the diagnosis
E. **True**

Q4

A. **True**
B. **False** – The radiograph is normal in most patients
C. **False** – PCO_2 is frequently decreased. Low arterial PO_2 is characteristic
D. **True** – The ventilated area is not perfused
E. **True** – This is particularly important in a patient with a DVT and recurrent pulmonary emboli

Q5

A. **True** – A premonitory sign is the discharge of slightly blood-stained serous fluid from the wound
B. **False** – It is rarely painful
C. **True** – Imperfect trimming, insertion or knotting of sutures can also be responsible
D. **True**
E. **True** – Conservative management results in an incisional hernia

Q6
A. **False** – Pre-operative breathing exercises decrease the incidence of pulmonary collapse. Adequate analgesia and treatment of existing respiratory disease are also preventative measures
B. **True**
C. **True**
D. **False** – Vigorous physiotherapy is the mainstay of treatment
E. **True** – Other treatments include adequate (but cautious) analgesia, humidified oxygen and antibiotics

Q7
A. **True** – Pre-operative breathing exercises, postoperative physiotherapy and stopping smoking reduce the risk
B. **False** – Spinal anaesthesia may reduce the incidence of atelectasis
C. **False** – Upper abdominal incisions are more likely to cause inadequate ventilation and atelectasis
D. **False** – Adequate analgesia reduces the risk
E. **True** – Smoking increases the risk and should therefore be stopped a few weeks prior to surgery

Q8
A. **True**
B. **True** – This complication is uncommon
C. **True** – The incidence is higher than during open cholecystectomy
D. **True** – Due to an incisional hernia at portal sites
E. **True** – e.g. when manipulating the porta hepatis

10. Trauma

Q1 **The clinical features of a tension pneumothorax include:**

A. Chest pain
B. Hypotension
C. Absent breath sounds on the affected side
D. Mediastinal shift towards the affected side
E. Decreased percussion resonance over the affected side

Q2 **The clinical features of cardiac tamponade are:**

A. Hypertension
B. Distended neck veins
C. Reduced heart sounds
D. Austin Flint murmur
E. Paradoxical chest movements

Q3 **Flail chest:**

A Is characterised by pulsus paradoxus
B. Complicates 20% of significant blunt thoracic trauma
C. Is usually treated with surgical stabilisation of the chest wall
D. Should be managed in an emergency by turning the patient onto the normal side
E. May be treated with epidural narcotics

Q4 **A complete division of the femoral nerve results in:**

A. Foot drop
B. Paraesthesia of the lateral aspect of the foot
C. Failure of knee extension
D. Sensory loss over the medial part of the lower leg
E. Failure of adduction of the thigh at the hip joint

Q5 **Injury to the ulnar nerve at the wrist results in:**

A. Wasting of the thenar eminence
B. Clawhand
C. Loss of the pincer-like action of the thumb and index finger
D. Sensory impairment over the palmar surface of the medial one and a half fingers
E. Wasting of the second lumbrical muscle

Q6 **Injury to the medial cord of the brachial plexus results in:**

A. Paralysis of all the intrinsic muscles of the hand
B. Loss of elbow flexion
C. Loss of cutaneous sensation over the anterior surface of the palm and fingers
D. Paralysis of the long flexors of the fingers
E. Paralysis of the pronator teres

Q7   Renal injuries:

A. Are caused by penetrating trauma in 85% of cases
B. Are managed conservatively in most cases
C. May cause hypertension
D. Associated with macroscopic haematuria should be investigated with intravenous urography (IVU)
E. Should be investigated with angiography if there is frank haematuria

Q8   Diagnostic peritoneal lavage in a trauma patient:

A. Is relatively contraindicated in pregnancy
B. Should be performed if there is unexplained shock
C. Is regarded as positive if the fluid red blood cell (RBC) count is $> 10\,000/mm^3$
D. Is regarded as positive if the fluid amylase level is 30 units
E. Has a high false-positive rate

Q9   The indications for thoracotomy following thoracic trauma include:

A. Haemothorax with initial drainage of 450 ml of blood
B. Haemothorax with bleeding at a rate of 200 ml/hour for 4 hours
C. Empyema
D. Cardiac tamponade
E. Flail chest with $PO_2 = 9\,kPa$ and $PCO_2 = 7\,kPa$

Q10   The acute blood loss of 1.5 litres leads to a decrease in:

A. The rate of oxygen extraction by peripheral tissues
B. The firing rate of carotid and aortic baroreceptors
C. Renin secretion
D. Peripheral vascular tone
E. Cardiac output

Q11   The following factors decrease cerebral blood flow (CBF):

A. Seizures
B. Inhalation of 7% CO_2
C. Intraventricular administration of norepinephrine
D. Chronic anaemia
E. Inhalation of hyperbaric oxygen

Q12   The spinothalamic tracts of the spinal cord transmit the following sensory modalities:

A. Pain
B. Two-point discrimination
C. Joint position
D. Temperature
E. Vibration

Q13 In a multiple trauma patient, computed tomography (CT):

A. Is more accurate than intravenous urography in detecting renal damage
B. Has a better pick-up rate if contrasts are used
C. Is more sensitive than peritoneal lavage in detecting small intraperitoneal bleeds
D. Shows fresh blood with a density of approximately 2 Hounsfield units
E. Of the head should be performed if the Glasgow coma score is 8 after resuscitation

Q14 The brain:

A. The brain receives 5% of the cardiac output
B. Blood flow to the brain is 800 ml/min
C. Intracranial pressure (ICP) is normally 0–10 mmHg
D. Intracranial pressure is directly proportional to the volume of skull contents
E. The brain compensates for initial rise in ICP by losing CSF in the lumbar thecal sac

Q15 Cervical spine radiographs:

A. Normally show a 4 mm atlanto-odontoid gap in adults
B. Open mouth odontoid views may show Jefferson fracture
C. Should always be taken in a multiple trauma patient
D. Swimmers view allows assessment of upper cervical vertebrae
E. Showing displacement > 50% of vertebral width usually indicate bilateral facet dislocation

Q16 The following are non-operative methods for reducing intracranial pressure:

A. Hypoventilation
B. Intravenous mannitol
C. The administration of atracurium
D. The administration of sodium nitroprusside
E   Placing the patient in the head-down position

Q17 Cerebral blood flow:

A. Accounts for about 15% of the cardiac output
B. Is decreased by hypocapnia
C. Is decreased by hypoxia
D. Is mainly controlled by sympathetic and parasympathetic mechanisms
E. Is increased by isoflurane in general anaesthesia

Q18 Consider the head CT scan of a trauma patient in Figure 10.1. The following statements are true:

A. M represents an extradural haematoma
B. N represents soft tissue swelling
C. A lumbar puncture is contraindicated in this patient
D. Hyperventilation should be avoided during the initial management
E. Urgent neurosurgery is indicated

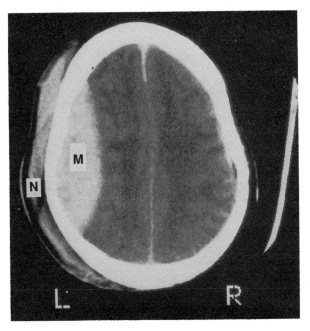

Figure 10.1

Q19   The clinical signs of pericardial tamponade include:

A. Loud heart sounds
B. Hypotension
C. Pulsus paradoxicus
D. Tachycardia
E. Reduced jugular venous pressure (JVP)

Q20   The clinical signs of spinal cord injury include:

A. Priapism
B. Decreased anal sphincter tone
C. Hypotension with relative tachycardia (assuming no significant blood loss)
D. Cullen's sign
E. Urinary retention

Q21   During intubation of a patient with a head injury:

A. It should be assumed that the patient has a cervical spine fracture
B. The intubating doctor must clearly visualise the vocal cords prior to intubation
C. Pressure on the cricoid cartilage must be avoided
D. A nasogastric tube should be passed in all cases
E. Tracheostomy is necessary if the intubation cannot be performed

Q22 The indications for endotracheal intubation in patients with severe head injuries include:

A. Absent gag reflex
B. Associated facial fracture
C. Raised intracranial pressure
D. $PaO_2 = 8\,kPa$ and $PaCO_2 = 6\,kPa$
E. Associated oropharyngeal bleeding

Q23 Signs of instability of the cervical spine include:

A. Bilateral facet dislocation
B. C1 posterior arch fracture
C. Angulation between vertebrae of 3°
D. Unilateral facet dislocation
E. Vertebral body compression by 10%

Q24 Compartment syndrome:

A. Is characterised by absent pulses
B. Often causes increasing pain
C. Does not develop in open fractures
D. Should be treated urgently with fasciotomy
E. Is characterised by a compartment pressure of 15–25 mmHg

Q25 The following signs and causative injuries are correctly paired:

A. Battle's sign – fracture of the mandibular condyle
B. Enophthalmos – fracture of the medial orbital wall
C. Bleeding from the middle ear – basal skull fracture
D. Subconjunctival ecchymosis – zygomatic fracture
E. CSF rhinorrhoea – basal skull fracture

Q26 Cervical injuries:

A. May be stabilised with halo traction
B. Associated with spinal cord injury may be treated with high-dose methyl-prednisolone
C. Requiring surgery should be operated on at least 24 hours after injury
D. May cause pupil constriction
E. Should be suspected if the retrotracheal space exceeds 6 mm in adults

Q27 The following cervical injuries are "stable":

A. "Teardrop" injury
B. Spinous process fracture
C. Jefferson fracture of C1
D. Hangman's fracture
E. C7 burst fracture

Q28 The acute blood loss of 1500 ml in an adult causes:

A. Thready tachycardia
B. Tachypnoea
C. A decrease in antidiuretic hormone (ADH) secretion
D. Metabolic alkalosis
E. The haemoglobin–oxygen dissociation curve to shift to the left

Q29 In the initial management of the burned patient:

A. Phenol burns should be placed under running water
B. IV fluid replacement is necessary in burns over > 15% of the body surface area
C. Tetanus prophylaxis is not necessary
D. Ringer's solution is to be preferred to human purified protein fraction (HPPF) in fluid resuscitation
E. Systemic antibiotics should be used routinely

Q30 The clinical features of Le Fort III maxillofacial fractures include:

A. Subconjunctival haemorrhage
B. CSF rhinorrhoea
C. A fracture line extending from the nasal bones into the medial orbital wall
D. Mobile maxilla
E. A transverse fracture line extending from above the alveolar ridge to the pterygoid region

Answers to Section 10

Q1
A. **True** – Due to lung collapse
B. **True** – Due to reduced venous return to the heart
C. **True**
D. **False** – The shift is to the opposite side
E. **False** – The percussion resonance is increased

Q2
A. **False** – Hypotension usually ensues
B. **True**
C. **True**
D. **False**
E. **False** – This is a feature of flail chest
Note: Cardiac tamponade is treated with urgent decompression by pericardiocentesis or via median sternotomy or left anterior thoracotomy

Q3
A. **False** – Paradoxical chest movement is characteristic
B. **True**
C. **False** – Skeletal fixation is not usually necessary owing to the availability of mechanical ventilation, which is the mainstay of treatment in patients with respiratory failure
D. **False** – The patient should be turned onto the affected side to stabilise the flail segment
E. **True**

Q4
A. **False** – This results from damage to the common peroneal nerve
B. **False** – This area is innervated by the common peroneal nerve
C. **True** – Due to paralysis of the quadriceps femoris
D. **True**
E. **False** – The adductors are supplied by the obturator nerve

Q5
A. **False** – This is a feature of median nerve injury
B. **True**
C. **False** – This is only slightly impaired owing to paralysis of the adductor pollicis
D. **True**
E. **False** – This muscle is supplied by the median nerve

Q6
A. **True**
B. **False**
C. **True**
D. **True**
E. **False** – This is supplied by the lateral head of the median nerve

Note: The medial cord branches include: (1) the medial head of the median nerve, (2) the ulnar nerve, (3) the medial pectoral nerve, (4) the medial cutaneous nerve of the arm and (5) the medial cutaneous nerve of the forearm

Q7
A. **False** – Blunt trauma accounts for 85% of cases
B. **True**
C. **True** – This is a long-term complication
D. **True**
E. **False** – Angiography is indicated if the kidney is not visualised on IVU

Q8
A. **True** – Morbid obesity and previous laparotomy are also relative contraindications
B. **True**
C. **False** – RBC > 100 000/mm³, white cell count > 500/mm³ and grossly blood-stained fluid indicate a positive lavage
D. **False** – Fluid amylase > 200 units is regarded as positive in peritoneal lavage
E. **False** – False-positive results are rare

Q9
A. **False** – Initial drainage > 1000 ml is an indication for thoracotomy
B. **True**
C. **True**
D. **True** – Sternotomy or left anterior thoracotomy may be required
E. **False** – Flail chest is usually managed with analgesia, physiotherapy and/or mechanical ventilation

Q10
A. **False** – This is increased
B. **True**
C. **False** – Renin secretion is increased in response to low renal perfusion due to hypovolaemia
D. **False** – The peripheral vascular tone increases to raise the blood pressure
E. **True** – The stroke volume falls

Q11
A. **False** – CBF increases
B. **False** – CBF increases by more than 100%
C. **False** – CBF increases
D. **False** – CBF increases
E. **True**

Q12
A. **True**
B. **False** – This travels in the posterior columns
C. **False** – This travels in the posterior columns
D. **True**
E. **False** – This travels in the posterior columns

62

Q13
A. **True** – It also gives faster results
B. **True**
C. **False** – Peritoneal lavage is more sensitive
D. **False** – It is approximately 24 Hounsfield units. The density decreases with time and reaches that of water at 72 hours
E. **True**

Q14
A. **False** – It receives 15%
B. **True**
C. **True**
D. **False**
E. **True**

Q15
A. **False** – The gap is 2.5 mm in adults and 4 mm in children
B. **True** – Of the atlas
C. **True** – Radiographs of the chest and pelvis should also be taken
D. **False** – The lower cervical vertebrae are shown in this view
E. **True**

Q16
A. **False** – Hyperventilation is used as the induced hypocapnia causes cerebral vasoconstriction and hence reduces cerebral blood flow
B. **True** – This is an osmotic diuretic that reduces the CSF volume and brain damage
C. **True** – This neuromuscular blocker relaxes muscles and hence reduces the intrathoracic pressure, which in turn lowers the venous pressure
D. **True** – This acts directly on the blood vessels producing the vasodilatation
E. **False** – The head-up position is used as it allows the pooling of venous blood in the dependent area

Q17
A. **True**
B. **True**
C. **False** – Hypoxia and hypercapnia increase cerebral blood flow
D. **False** – Autonomic mechanisms seem to be unimportant
E. **True**

Q18
A. **True**
B. **True**
C. **True** – Lumbar puncture could precipitate coning
D. **False** – Hyperventilation, steroids and mannitol help to reduce raised intracranial pressure
E. **True** – To evacuate the haematoma

Q19
A. **False** – The heart sounds become muffled
B. **True**
C. **True**
D. **True**
E. **False** – JVP is usually raised. Beck's triad consists of raised JVP, muffled heart sounds and hypotension

Q20
A. **True** – The penis does not have to be fully erect to diagnose this
B. **True**
C. **False** – Hypotension with relative bradycardia may result from interruption of sympathetic outflow
D. **False** – This is a sign of pancreatitis (bruising in the peri-umbilical area)
E. **True**

Q21
A. **True** – The neck should be immobilised
B. **False** – Experienced anaesthetists are able to intubate without visualising the cords clearly
C. **False** – Such a manoeuvre may reduce the incidence of aspiration
D. **False** – This is contraindicated in basal skull fractures
E. **True**

Q22
A. **True**
B. **False**
C. **True** – To allow hyperventilation
D. **True**
E. **True** – To protect the airway

Q23
A. **False** – This is a stable fracture
B. **True**
C. **False** – Angulation > 10° indicates instability
D. **False** – Bilateral facet dislocation indicates instability
E. **False** – Compression > 25% indicates instability

Q24
A. **False** – The presence of pulses does not exclude this syndrome
B. **True**
C. **False** – An incidence of 15% has been reported
D. **True**
E. **False** – The compartment pressure usually exceeds 30 mmHg

Q25
A. **False** – Middle cranial fossa fractures may cause a positive Battle's sign (bruising behind the ear)
B. **True**
C. **True**
D. **True**
E. **True**

Q26
A. **True**
B. **True** – 30 mg/kg IV infusion over 15 minutes as early as possible, then 5.4 mg/kg for 23 hours
C. **False**
D. **True** – Due to interruption of sympathetic innervation
E. **False** – The retrotracheal space is < 20 mm and the retropharyngeal space < 6 mm in normal adults

Q27
A. **False** – This is unstable
B. **True**
C. **False**
D. **False** – Hangman's fracture is traumatic spondylolisthesis of C2
E. **True**

Q28
A. **True** – Due to catecholamine release
B. **True** – Due to hypoxia and acidosis
C. **False** – ADH output increases to compensate for hypovolaemia
D. **False** – Metabolic acidosis ensues
E. **False** – The curve shifts to the right to release oxygen readily for hypoxic tissue

Q29
A. **False** – Water accelerates the absorption of this chemical
B. **True** – IV fluids are required for burns over > 15% in adults and > 10% in children
C. **False** – Should be given as indicated
D. **False** – HPPF is to be preferred
E. **False** – Routine use encourages the emergence of resistant strains

Q30
A. **True**
B. **True**
C. **False** – This is true of a Le Fort II fracture
D. **True** – The central third of the face is detached from the cranial base in Le Fort fractures
E. **False** – This is true of Le Fort I fractures

11. Head and Neck

Q1   **Tongue cancer:**

A. Thickness is the best single predictor of prognosis
B. Often causes earache
C. Of the posterior third has a better prognosis
D. Of the anterior third is treated with partial glossectomy
E. Treatment may necessitate laryngectomy

Q2   **Lip cancer:**

A. Affects the lower lip in 93% of cases
B. At the angle of the mouth has a better prognosis than at the lower lip
C. At the angle of the mouth is commonly treated with radiotherapy
D. Involving the mental nerve has a 5 year survival rate of 75%
E. > 2 cm in size is usually treated with surgical excision and plastic reconstruction

Q3   **The complications of tracheostomy include:**

A. Surgical emphysema
B. Granuloma of the vocal cords
C. Air embolism
D. Fat embolism
E. Tracheal stenosis

Q4   **Considering the thyroid gland:**

A. It arises from the same branchial pouch as the upper parathyroid glands
B. It is separated from the strap muscles by the pretracheal fascia
C. The middle thyroid veins course laterally to drain into the internal jugular vein
D. The gland arises at the foramen caecum
E. In thyroidectomy the recurrent laryngeal nerve is frequently damaged when the superior thyroid artery is ligated

Q5   **In radical neck dissection, the following structures are usually removed:**

A. Submandibular gland
B. Internal carotid artery
C. Internal jugular vein
D. Lipuinal nerve
E. Cervical sympathetic chain

Q6   **The indications for tracheostomy include:**

A. Temporary airway control in acute head injuries
B. Flail chest
C. Tetanus
D. Carcinoma of the tongue
E. Prolonged endotracheal intubation

Q7   Laryngeal carcinoma:

A. Is associated with cigarette smoking in most cases
B. Presents with hoarseness as the commonest symptom
C. In situ is treated with mucosal stripping
D. Stage T1 is usually treated with total laryngectomy and neck dissection
E. Is radioresistant

Q8   Maxillary sinus carcinoma:

A. Is adenocarcinoma in most cases
B. May present with proptosis and diplopia
C. Is radioresistant
D. Stage T1 is treated with maxillectomy
E. Stage T3 is treated with pre-operative radiotherapy followed by surgical resection

Q9   The parotid gland:

A. Is divided into superficial and deep parts by the facial nerve
B. Duct passes forward deep to the masseter muscle
C. Is enclosed in a dense fibrous capsule
D. Receives parasympathetic secretomotor fibres via the great auricular nerve
E. Glenoid process extends medially behind the temporomandibular joint

Q10   The palatine tonsil:

A. Is separated from the superior constrictor muscle by lax connective tissue
B. Receives blood supply from the facial artery
C. Lies anterior to the palatoglossal arch
D. Is separated from the glossopharyngeal nerve by the superior constrictor muscle of the pharynx
E. Receives blood supply from the ascending pharyngeal artery

Q11   About the thyroid:

A. The gland selectively concentrates iodine from plasma iodide
B. Thyroid stimulating hormone (TSH) is secreted by acidophil cells in the anterior pituitary gland
C. Gland vascularity and cellularity is increased by TSH
D. Thyroxine (T4) has a half-life of 12 hours
E. T4 produces effects within 6 hours of secretion

Q12   Carbimazole:

A. Is concentrated in the thyroid gland within minutes of administration
B. Usually renders a thyrotoxic patient euthyroid within one week of therapy
C. Is contraindicated in pregnancy
D. May produce leucopenia
E. May be combined with thyroxine in the treatment of thyrotoxicosis

Q13 Salivary calculi:

A. Consist of calcium oxalate in most cases
B. Are commonest in the parotid gland
C. Commonly cause sialadenitis
D. Near the end of the duct can be removed transorally
E. Frequently necessitate excision of the gland involved

Q14 Epistaxis from Little's area may be treated with:

A. Cotton wool soaked in 5% cocaine and 1/1000 adrenaline
B. Digital pressure over the nasal bones
C. Digital pressure over the lower nose
D. Silver nitrate crystals fused to a wire
E. Cotton wool soaked in phentolamine

Q15 Pleomorphic adenoma of the parotid:

A. Is the commonest tumour affecting the gland
B. Contains cartilage
C. Has a true capsule
D. Usually affects the superficial part of the gland
E. Is usually treated with wide total parotidectomy

Q16 Acute otitis media:

A. Of bacterial origin is most commonly caused by *Staphylococcus aureus*
B. Symptoms may improve with myringotomy
C. Is a recognised cause of subdural abscesses
D. In children under the age of 5 years should be treated with penicillin
E. Complications include mastoiditis

Q17 Acute (closed angle) glaucoma:

A. Is a recognised cause of red eye
B. Is characterised by a small pupil
C. Can be treated with laser iridectomy
D. Is characterised by normal visual acuity
E. Can be treated with topical pilocarpine

Answers to Section 11

Q1
A. **True** – Lesions thicker than 1 cm have a poor prognosis
B. **True** – This may be due to referred pain from the lingual branch of the trigeminal nerve via the auriculotemporal branch
C. **False** – The prognosis is worse
D. **True**
E. **True** – Posterior tongue lesions may invade the preglottic space

Q2
A. **True** – 5% affect the upper lip and 2% affect the angle of the mouth
B. **False** – This location has a worse prognosis
C. **True**
D. **False** – Involvement of the mental nerve is associated with a high incidence of lymph node metastases and 46% survival at 5 years
E. **True**

Q3
A. **True**
B. **True**
C. **True**
D. **False**
E. **True** – Other complications include dislodgement of the tube, haemorrhage, obstruction of the tube or trachea, and sepsis

Q4
A. **False**
B. **True**
C. **True** – This is the first vessel to be encountered in thyroidectomy
D. **True** – It arises at the base of the tongue and migrates downwards
E. **False** – The external laryngeal nerve is closely related to the superior thyroid artery, whereas the recurrent laryngeal nerve may be closely related to the inferior thyroid artery

Q5
A. **True**
B. **False**
C. **True** – Because the deep cervical lymph nodes are closely attached to it
D. **False**
E. **False**

Q6
A. **False** – Endotracheal intubation provides temporary airway control
B. **True**
C. **True**
D. **True**
E. **True**

Q7
A. **True** – Significant smoking history is obtained in > 90% of cases
B. **True** – Other symptoms include haemoptysis, stridor and dysphagia
C. **True** – Or radiotherapy
D. **False** – T1 lesions can be treated with radiotherapy or hemilaryngectomy. The 5 year survival rate (for T1) is approximately 87%
E. **False** – It responds to radiotherapy

Q8
A. **False** – Squamous cell carcinoma is the commonest
B. **True** – Due to upward extension
C. **False** – It is radiosensitive
D. **True** – Radiotherapy may be required for positive resection margins or recurrence
E. **True** – Orbital exenteration and skin excision may be performed when indicated

Q9
A. **True**
B. **False** – The duct passes superficial to the masseter. This makes it susceptible to damage in facial injuries
C. **True** – This limits the swelling in parotitis
D. **False** – It receives these fibres via the auriculotemporal nerve. In Frey's syndrome the injured auriculotemporal nerve joins the distal end of the great auricular nerve that supplies the sweat glands in the facial skin
E. **True**

Q10
A. **True**
B. **True**
C. **False** – It lies posterior to the palatoglossal arch
D. **True** – The nerve supplies the tonsil
E. **True**

Q11
A. **True**
B. **False** – It is secreted by basophil cells
C. **True**
D. **False** The $t_{1/2}$ of T4 is 6–7 days. Therefore it cannot be administered more frequently than once daily
E. **False** – Maximal activity of T4 is not reached until 7–10 days after administration (compared with 24 hours for T3, which is more valuable in the emergency treatment of myxoedema coma)

Q12
A. **False** – This is true of methimazole
B. **False** – This takes 1–4 months
C. **False**
D. **True**
E. **True** – To prevent hypothyroidism and provide a finer control

Q13
A. **False** – Calcium carbonate and phosphate stones are the commonest
B. **False** – The submandibular gland with its long tortuous duct is the commonest site
C. **True**
D **True**
E. **True** – Multiple deep stones causing symptoms require excision of the gland

Q14
A. **True**
B. **False** – This is ineffective
C. **True**
D. **True** – Electric cautery or diathermy may also be used
E. **False** – Phentolamine is an α-blocker, which causes vasodilatation

Q15
A. **True**
B. **False** – The blue staining mucus looks like cartilage
C. **False** – The capsule is a false one, hence the high recurrence rate following excision
D. **True**
E. **False** – Conservative partial parotidectomy is used

Q16
A. **False** – *Pneumococcus* and *Haemophilus influenzae* are the commonest bacterial causes
B. **True** – Pain and fever improve with myringotomy
C. **True**
D. **False** – *Haemophilus influenzae* is the commonest cause in this age group, therefore amoxycillin is to be preferred
E. **True**

Q17
A. **True**
B. **False** – The pupil is usually large
C. **True**
D. **False** – The visual acuity is usually reduced
E. **True** – This is a cholinergic drug

12. Oncology

Q1 **The following factors facilitate metastasis of cancer cells:**

A. Metalloproteinase inhibitors
B. Loss of E-cadherin expression
C. Angiogenesis peptides
D. CD8+ T cells
E. Integrin expression

Q2 **The consequences of radiotherapy include:**

A. Endarteritis obliterans
B. Development of a second malignancy
C. Gastrointestinal fistulae
D. Promotion of tumour angiogenesis
E. Mucositis

Q3 **The following are recognised chemical carcinogens in humans:**

A. Aflatoxin
B. Omeprazole
C. Blue asbestos
D. β-Naphthylamine
E. 5-Aminosalicylate

Q4 **With reference to the process of metastasis of malignant cells, the following statements are true:**

A. Metastases may appear 25 years following surgical clearance of primary tumour
B. The presence of metalloproteinase decreases the tumour's ability to invade
C. The absence of regional lymph node involvement excludes metastases to distant organs
D. Micrometastases in the circulation may be destroyed by host defences
E. Sarcomas tend to spread via the lymphatic system

Q5 **Ionising radiation:**

A. Damages cellular DNA
B. Is more effective in hypoxic tumour cells
C. Is more effective during the G2 phase of the cell cycle
D. Maximal permissible dose for medical staff is 2 cGy per year
E. Dosage in grays measures energy absorbed

Q6   Oestrogen receptors:

A. Are cytoplasmic proteins
B. Can be detected using monoclonal antibody H222
C. Are markers of more aggressive malignant behaviour
D. Are present in 60% of ductal carcinoma *in situ* (DCIS) lesions
E. May be absent in breast carcinoma, and this excludes tamoxifen as a treatment

Q7   A 1 cm malignant tumour:

A. Contains approximately 10^9 cells
B. Usually results from 10 doublings
C. Usually exhibits cellular heterogeneity
D. Has cells that are more strongly attached to one another than those in a similar benign tumour
E. May show a Gompertzian growth pattern as it increases in size

Q8   Tumours in which cure is possible with chemotherapy include:

A. Melanoma
B. Testicular teratoma
C. Hodgkin's lymphoma
D. Colorectal carcinoma
E. Hypernephroma

Q9   The following cancers (caused by inherited mutations) and locations of causative gene are correctly paired:

A. Breast carcinoma (*BRCA-1*) – 17q21
B. Retinoblastoma (*RB1*) – 17p13
C. Colorectal carcinoma (*APC*) – 5q21
D. Sarcoma (*p53*) – 13q14
E. Medullary thyroid carcinoma (*RET*) – 10q11

Q10   Malignant skin melanoma:

A. Arises in a pre-existing mole in approximately 40% of melanoma cases
B. Of the superficial spreading type is the commonest
C. Has a better prognosis in males
D. Stage IIb is treated with surgical excision and block dissection of regional nodes
E. Prognosis is independent of Clark's level

Q11   The following are recognised growth suppressor genes:

A. *BRCA-1*
B. *p53*
C. *c-myc*
D. *bcl2*
E. *h-ras*

Q12 Epstein–Barr virus (EBV) has been implicated in the aetiology of the following cancers:

A. Colorectal carcinoma
B. Cervical carcinoma
C. Hepatocellular carcinoma
D. Breast carcinoma
E. Nasopharyngeal carcinoma

Q13 Interferon-2:

A. Has antiviral activity
B. Is a recognised cause of bone marrow suppression
C. Is licensed for use in breast cancer
D. Is licensed for use in advanced renal cell carcinoma
E. May cause remission of Kaposi's sarcoma

Q14 Interleukin-2:

A. Stimulates T-cell growth and activation
B. Is a glycoprotein
C. Has direct anti-tumour effects
D. Has a response rate of 75% in renal cell cancer
E. Can be given safely to outpatients

Q15 Tumour necrosis factor:

A. Is a mediator of endotoxin-induced shock
B. Is a cytokine
C. Decreases interleukin-2 (IL-2) receptor synthesis by T cells
D. Has been used in the treatment of malignant melanoma
E. Is not neurotoxic

Q16 Oncogenes:

A. Are genes capable of causing cancer
B. Have been isolated for about 50% of human cancers
C. Code for protein kinases in about 50% of viral oncogenes
D. May uncouple the intranuclear mechanisms involved in growth control from the need for an external stimulus
E. Include growth suppressor genes

Q17 Figure 12.1 represents different phases of the cell cycle. The following statements are correct:

A. Cells are most sensitive to ionising radiation during the S phase
B. DNA synthesis is confined to the S phase
C. During the G1 phase, the cells are metabolically inactive
D. The total duration of the cell cycle in normal tissues is constant
E. The cells of solid tumours in humans proceed through the cell cycle in the same phase

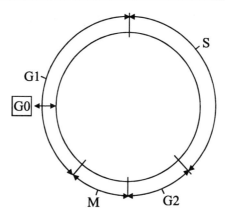

Figure 12.1   The cell cycle

Q18   The following tumour markers and malignancies are correctly paired:

A. α-Fetoprotein – hepatocellular carcinoma
B. CA19-9 – testicular teratoma
C. Carcino-embryonic antigen (CEA) – colorectal carcinoma
D. Calcitonin – follicular carcinoma of the thyroid
E. Human chorionic gonadotrophin (hCG) – breast carcinoma

Answers to Section 12

Q1
A. **False** – Metalloproteinase secreted by adjacent fibroblasts destroys surrounding tissue barriers
B. **True** – This leads to loss of cell-to-cell cohesion
C. **True** – They mediate neovascularisation
D. **False** – These cells destroy tumour cells
E. **True** – This assists metastatic cell arrest in the target organs

Q2
A. **True** – This may result in ischaemia of the organ involved
B. **True**
C. **True** – Enteritis, intra-abdominal adhesions and enteric strictures are also recognised sequelae
D. **False**
E. **True**

Q3
A. **True** – Hepatic carcinoma
B. **False** – There is no evidence
C. **True** – Mesothelioma of pleura and peritoneum, and pulmonary carcinoma
D. **True** – Bladder carcinoma
E. **False** – Aspirin may have a role in preventing colorectal cancer

Q4
A. **True** – This feature is encountered in breast cancer
B. **False** – Metalloproteinase facilitates local invasion and distant spread
C. **False** – Micrometastases commonly occur before regional node metastases
D. **True** – Only a small proportion of micrometastases survive as secondary metastases
E. **False** – Sarcomas tend to metastasise via the blood stream

Q5
A. **True** – This is the main mechanism of action
B. **False** – Hypoxic cells are radioresistant
C. **False** – It is more effective during the S and late G1 phases
D. **True** – This dosage does not seem to increase the incidence of cancer among hospital staff
E. **True** – 1 Gy = 1 J/kg

Q6
A. **False** – They are nuclear proteins
B. **True**
C. **False** – The presence of oestrogen receptors indicates a less aggressive behaviour and a better prognosis
D. **False** – Oestrogen receptors are present in 60% of invasive cancers and 30% of DCIS lesions
E. **False** – Tamoxifen is effective (although to a lesser extent) in oestrogen-receptor-negative breast cancers

Q7

A. **True**

B. **False** – It results from 30–50 doublings

C. **True** – The cells are monoclonal initially, but they become heterogeneous due to mutations

D. **False** – There is less cellular cohesion in malignancy

E. **True** – In this growth pattern, the growth rate decreases as size increases

Q8

A. **False**

B. **True**

C. **True**

D. **False**

E. **False**

Q9

A. **True**

B. **False** – The *RB1* location is 13q14

C. **True**

D. **False** – The *p53* location is 17p13

E. **True**

Q10

A. **True**

B. **True** – 65% of cases

C. **False** – Females have a better prognosis

D. **True**

E. **False** – The higher the level, the worse the prognosis

Q11

A. **True** – This is a breast cancer gene

B. **True**

C. **False** – This cellular proto-oncogene is involved in the control of the cell cycle

D. **False** – This is an anti-apoptosis gene

E. **False** – This cellular proto-oncogene is involved in signal transduction

Q12

A. **False**

B. **False** – This is associated with human papilloma virus and herpes simplex virus

C. **False** – This is associated with hepatitis B and C

D. **False**

E. **True** – Burkitt's lymphoma has also been linked to EBV

Q13

A. **True**

B. **True** – Other side effects include hypotension, flu-like illness, nausea and vomiting

C. **False**

D. **True** – The response rate is 15%

E. **True** – The other indications include multiple myeloma, non-Hodgkin's lymphoma, hairy cell leukaemia and chronic myeloid leukaemia

Q14
A. **True**
B. **True**
C. **False** – It acts indirectly
D. **False** – The response rate is 12%
E. **True**

Q15
A. **True**
B. **True**
C. **False** – It activates B cells and increases IL-2 receptor synthesis by T cells
D. **True** – It has been used in isolated limb perfusion leading to impressive regression of advanced malignant melanoma
E. **False**

Q16
A. **True**
B. **False** – They have been isolated for only 15%
C. **True**
D. **True**
E. **False** – Growth suppressor factors are anti-oncogenes

Q17
A. **False** – They are most sensitive during the M and G2 phases
B. **True**
C. **False** – They are active, synthesising RNA and proteins
D. **False** – This is true of malignant tumours
E. **False** – This is true of experimental tumours

Q18
A. **True** – High serum levels are found in about 70% of cases
B. **False** – CA19-9 is a marker for pancreatic carcinoma
C. **True**
D. **False** –The calcitonin level may increase in medullary carcinoma of the thyroid
E. **False** – hCG rises in choriocarcinoma, causing a falsely positive pregnancy test in males with testicular carcinoma

13. Vascular Surgery

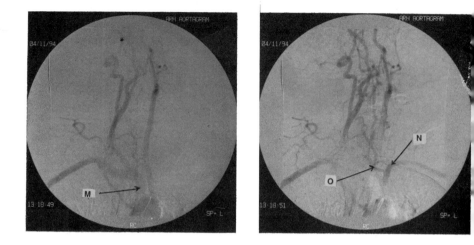

Figure 13.1 (a) Arch aortogram. (b) Arch aortogram (later film)

Q1 **Consider the arch aortograms in Figure 13.1. The following statements are true:**

A. M is the right brachiocephalic artery
B. N is the left subclavian artery
C. N is directly perfused from the aortic arch
D. O is the left common carotid artery
E. The angiogram suggests the diagnosis of subclavian steal syndrome

Q2 **A 65-year-old man presented with a tender abdominal mass. Computed tomography was performed (Figure 13.2). The following are true:**

A. M is a paravertebral muscle
B. N is the left rectus abdominis muscle
C. This patient has a right renal mass
D. The abdominal aorta appears normal
E. Urgent surgical intervention is indicated

Q3 **Occlusive disease of the femoral artery:**

A. Most commonly presents with calf claudication
B. May cause Leriche's syndrome
C. Usually occurs at the level of the adductor hiatus
D. Can be treated with percutaneous transluminal angioplasty (PTA) if the occlusion is complete
E. Symptoms improve with nifedipine

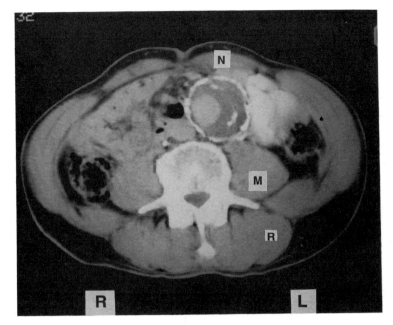

Figure 13.2   Computed tomography of the abdomen

Q4   The great saphenous vein:

A. Passes behind the medial malleolus
B. Joins the femoral vein about 3.5 cm below and lateral to the pubic tubercle
C. Usually lies behind the superficial external pudendal artery
D. Receives fewer tributaries than the femoral vein at the level of the saphenous opening
E. Has more deep perforators below the knee than in the thigh

Q5   The abdominal aorta:

A. Pierces the diaphragm in front of the T12 vertebra
B. Divides into two common iliac arteries at the level of the L4 vertebra
C. Gives off five lumbar arteries on both sides
D. Is closely related to the left sympathetic trunk
E. Aneurysms usually arise above the origins of the renal arteries

Q6   The internal jugular vein:

A. Begins at the jugular foramen as a continuation of the sigmoid sinus
B. Passes behind the thoracic duct on the left side
C. Runs alongside the chain of deep cervical lymph nodes
D. Lies medial to the internal carotid artery within the carotid sheath
E. Passes anterior to the phrenic nerve

Q7   Consequences of lower limb reperfusion following acute ischaemia include:

A. Decrease in serum creatine phosphokinase (CPK) levels
B. Metabolic alkalosis
C. Myoglobinuria
D. Acute tubular necrosis
E. Rise in intracompartment pressure of the calf compartment

Q8   Inflammatory aortic aneurysms:

A. Account for approximately 40% of all abdominal aortic aneurysms
B. Have a thicker wall
C. Should be treated with corticosteroids before surgery
D. Involve an inflammatory process that does not resolve after surgical repair
E. Are frequently adherent to the duodenum

Q9   Popliteal artery aneurysm:

A. Is the commonest peripheral aneurysm
B. Is rarely bilateral
C. Thrombosis may be treated with intra-arterial streptokinase
D. Is caused by atherosclerosis in most cases
E. Is rarely associated with other proximal aneurysms

Q10   The inferior vena cava (IVC):

A. Is formed by the two common iliac veins anterior to the right common iliac artery
B. Pierces the diaphragm at the level of the T12 vertebra
C. Directly receives the left suprarenal vein
D. Is closely related to the right sympathetic trunk
E. Receives the two hepatic veins

Q11   The long saphenous vein (LSV) usually receives the following tributaries in the femoral triangle:

A. The superficial epigastric vein
B. The deep circumflex iliac vein
C. The deep external pudendal vein
D. The lateral accessory vein
E. The superficial circumflex iliac vein

Q12   Ruptured abdominal aortic aneurysm:

A. Has a 50% mortality rate
B. Diagnosis should be confirmed by computed tomography
C. Is usually repaired with a woven Dacron® graft
D. Wall is usually used to cover the synthetic graft
E. Raises serum amylase

Q13   Aorto-iliac occlusive disease:

A. Is a recognised cause of impotence
B. May present with a gangrenous toe
C. Treatment with axillofemoral bypass has a greater patency rate than aortobifemoral bypass
D. Causing complete occlusion can be treated with percutaneous transluminal angioplasty (PTA)
E. May be treated with femorofemoral crossover graft in the unfit patient

Q14   The management of reperfusion syndrome following a successful re-vascularisation of an acutely ischaemic lower limb includes:

A. Calf fasciotomy
B. Haemodialysis
C. Acid forced diuresis
D. Mannitol
E. Bicarbonate

Q15   Femoral artery aneurysm:

A. Is commoner than abdominal aortic aneurysm (AAA)
B. Is usually inflammatory in origin
C. Should be investigated with angiography
D. Surgical treatment involves exclusion of the aneurysm from the circulation with ligation and graft bypass
E. Is a recognised cause of distal emboli

Q16   Autogenous vein grafts:

A. Have a greater thrombogenicity potential than synthetic vascular grafts
B. Are easier to revise than synthetic vascular grafts
C. Have a greater patency rate at 5 years than synthetic vascular grafts
D. May be complicated by intimal hyperplasia
E. Undergo spasm when exposed to papaverine

Q17   Unfractionated heparin:

A. May cause thrombocytopenia
B. Anticoagulation is best monitored by measuring the international normalised ratio (INR)
C. Is antagonised by protamine sulphate
D. Has a longer duration of action than low molecular weight heparin
E. Is usually given as 5000 units subcutaneously twice daily to treat an established deep vein thrombosis

Q18   Causes of Raynaud's phenomenon include:

A. Scleroderma
B. Cryoglobulinaemia
C. Horner's syndrome
D. Phentolamine
E. Vibrating tools

Q19 Dissecting aneurysms of the aorta:

A. Usually arise because of cystic medial necrosis
B. Start in the descending aorta in most cases
C. Have an increased incidence in Marfan's syndrome
D. May cause electromechanical dissociation of the electrocardiogram (ECG)
E. Are usually accompanied by ECG changes suggestive of myocardial infarction (MI)

Q20 The following are recognised causes of mycotic aneurysms:

A. *Mycobacterium tuberculosis*
B. *Staphylococcus aureus*
C. Marfan's syndrome
D. *Salmonella*
E. *Trichophyton rubrum*

Q21 Dacron vascular grafts:

A. Of the woven variety should be preclotted prior to use
B. Are made of polytetrafluoroethylene (PTFE)
C. Are the grafts of choice for aortobifemoral bypass
D. Are the synthetic grafts of choice for femoropopliteal bypass
E. May be coated with albumin

Q22 The following are recognised complications of aortic aneurysm repair:

A. Paraplegia
B. Melaena
C. Impotence
D. Adult respiratory distress syndrome
E. Trash foot

Q23 Renal artery stenosis:

A. Due to fibromuscular dysplasia is more common in men
B. Increases renin output from the affected kidney
C. May be treated with percutaneous transluminal angioplasty
D. Should be treated medically in children
E. Due to fibromuscular dysplasia has a poor prognosis

Q24 Aortic graft infection:

A. Is usually caused by streptococci
B. May occur many years after surgery
C. Is frequently caused by *Helicobacter pylori*
D. Incidence is significantly reduced by peri-operative antibiotics
E. Rarely requires surgical treatment

Q25 Treatments for Raynaud's disease include:

A. β-Blockers
B. Nifedipine
C. Ergot
D. Cervical sympathectomy
E. Naftidrofuryl oxalate

Q26 Abdominal aortic aneurysms:

A. Are caused by atherosclerosis in most cases
B. Usually expand at 1 cm in diameter per year
C. Measuring 4.5–7 cm in diameter have a 5 year rupture rate of 35%
D. May be caused by *Salmonella*
E. Greater than 7 cm in diameter have a 5 year rupture rate of 45%

Q27 Recognised complications of sclerotherapy for varicose veins include:

A. Skin ulceration
B. Sudeck's dystrophy
C. Deep venous thrombosis
D. Madura foot
E. Brown pigmentation of the skin

Q28 The clinical features of the postphlebitic limb include:

A. Trash foot
B. Branham's sign
C. Hyperpigmentation of the skin
D. Venous claudication
E. Pain relieved by placing the limb in the dependent position

Q29 The clinical features of thoracic outlet compression syndrome include:

A. Oedema of the arm
B. Cyanosis of the arm
C. Paraesthesia over the medial fingers
D. Gangrene of the fingers
E. Carpal tunnel compression syndrome

Q30 The management of thoracic outlet syndrome (TOS) includes:

A. Thoracic sympathectomy
B. Excision of the first rib
C. Excision of the cervical intervertebral disc
D. Excision of the cervical rib
E. Division of the scalenus anterior

Q31   Recognised treatments for chronic lymphoedema include:

A. Excision of skin and subcutaneous tissue
B. Le Veen shunt
C. Thompson procedure
D. Compression stockings
E. McCash procedure

Q32   Primary lymphoedema:

A. Is most commonly caused by Milroy's disease
B. Is commoner in females
C. May be caused by *Wuchereria bancrofti*
D. Usually presents in the first decade
E. Frequently causes skin ulceration

Q33   The clinical features of the diabetic foot include:

A. Clawing of the toes
B. Charcot arthropathy
C. Medial calcification of small arteries
D. Response of skin changes to sympathectomy
E. Painful skin ulcers over the heel

Q34   Buerger's disease:

A. Has equal sex distribution
B. Characteristically involves the medium-sized arteries of the extremities
C. Is a panarteritis
D. Will stabilise if the patient stops smoking
E. Causes foot claudication

Q35   Varicose veins:

A. Are the commonest cause of venous ulceration
B. Have a higher incidence in multiparous women
C. May be treated using sclerotherapy with thrombin
D. Are usually caused by a reduced number of venous valves
E. May become calcified

Q36   Carotid endarterectomy:

A. Can be performed under local anaesthesia
B. If successful, reduces the risk of ipsilateral stroke by 70%
C. Must include an intra-arterial shunt to protect the cerebral circulation during arterial clamping
D. May be complicated by hypoglossal nerve palsy
E. Has an operative mortality rate of approximately 10%

Q37 The indications for carotid endarterectomy in patients with carotid stenosis include:

A. A complete stroke
B. Stroke in evolution
C. 50% stenosis without symptoms
D. 75% stenosis with a recent transient ischaemic attack
E. Amaurosis fugax with 75% stenosis

Q38 Absolute predictors of healing in below-knee amputation include:

A. Calf Doppler pressure > 30 mmHg
B. Transcutaneous PO_2 > 40 mmHg
C. Absence of gangrene above the ankle
D. Absence of sensory loss below the knee
E. None of the above

Q39 The complications of below-knee amputation include:

A. Neuroma of the posterior tibial nerve
B. Aneurysm of the popliteal artery
C. Phantom pain
D. Knee joint contractures
E. Gas gangrene

Q40 The contraindications to below-knee amputation include:

A. A transcutaneous PO_2 of 45 mmHg
B. Severe osteoarthritis of the knee joint
C. Impalpable dorsalis pedis pulse
D. Paralysis of the leg (to be amputated) due to a previous cerebrovascular accident
E. Sensory neuropathy affecting the future stump

Q41 Foot ulcers secondary to arterial insufficiency may be treated with:

A. Elevation of the affected leg
B. Antibiotics
C. Debridement of necrotic tissue
D. Femorotibial bypass
E. Compressive stockings

Q42 Cystic hygromas:

A. Are the least common benign tumours of the lymphatics
B. Occur most commonly in the neck
C. May occur in the groin
D. In the neck should be excised
E. Should be excised completely even if cranial nerves are sacrificed

Q43 A 65-year-old man presents with left calf claudication (claudication distance 20 m). Angiography demonstrates total occlusion of the left superficial femoral artery. Appropriate treatments include:

A. Percutaneous transluminal angioplasty
B. Femoropopliteal bypass using a reversed long saphenous vein (LSV) graft
C. Femorotibial bypass using an LSV graft *in situ*
D. Femorofemoral crossover bypass using a GORE-TEX® graft
E. Atenolol to vasodilate the muscle vasculature

Answers to Section 13

Q1
A. **True**
B. **True**
C. **False** – It is perfused by retrograde filling via the left vertebral artery, O
D. **False** – O is the left vertebral artery
E. **True** – The subclavian artery is occluded just distal to its origin

Q2
A. **False** – M is a psoas muscle. The paravertebral muscles are designated R
B. **True**
C. **False**
D. **False** – The aorta appears aneurysmal with double calcification shadow in its wall suggestive of previous dissection
E. **True** – A tender aortic aneurysm should be repaired urgently

Q3
A. **True**
B. **False** – This may be caused by aorto-iliac disease (buttock and thigh claudication and impotence)
C. **True**
D. **False** – Short incomplete occlusions may be treated with PTA
E. **False** – This calcium channel blocker reduces blood flow

Q4
A. **False** – It passes in front of the medial malleolus
B. **True**
C. **False** – It usually lies in front of this artery but may lie behind it
D. **False** – It has more numerous tributaries at this level and this fact helps to distinguish it from the femoral vein during surgery
E. **True**

Q5
A. **True**
B. **True**
C. **False** – It gives rise to four lumbar arteries
D. **True**
E. **False** – They arise below the level of the renal arteries in most cases

Q6
A. **True**
B. **False** – It passes in front of the thoracic duct
C. **True**
D. **False** – It lies lateral to the internal carotid artery
E. **True**

Q7
A. **False** – Serum CPK rise is due to rhabdomyolysis
B. **False** – Acidosis ensues
C. **True**
D. **True**
E. **True**

Q8
A. **False** – They account for 5–10% of cases
B. **True** – Due to inflammation
C. **False** – There is no evidence that this is beneficial
D. **False** – Surgery usually results in resolution of the inflammatory process
E. **True** – It is advisable to avoid dissecting the aneurysm off the duodenum to avoid accidental duodenotomy

Q9
A. **True**
B. **False** – It is bilateral in approximately 35% of cases
C. **True**
D. **True**
E. **False** – Abdominal aortic aneurysms are often associated with popliteal aneurysms

Q10
A. **False** – It is formed behind the right common iliac artery
B. **False** – It pierces the diaphragm at the level of the T8 vertebra
C. **False** – The suprarenal vein feeds into the IVC via the renal vein
D. **True** – The trunk lies behind the right border of the IVC
E. **True**

Q11
A. **True**
B. **False**
C. **True**
D. **True**
E. **True**
Note: Figure 13.3 illustrates the tributaries of the LSV in the femoral triangle

Q12
A. **True**
B. **False** – Investigations should not delay surgical intervention
C. **True**
D. **True** – This may reduce the incidence of aorto-enteric fistula and graft infection
E. **True** – The serum amylase may be moderately raised

Q13
A. **True**
B. **True** – Due to distal embolisation
C. **False** – Aortobifemoral bypass is superior (5 year patency rate = 85%). In the unfit patient less radical procedures, such as axillofemoral and femorofemoral bypass, are reasonable surgical options
D. **False** – PTA is indicated for short stenosis and in the absence of complete occlusion
E. **True** – This may be performed under local, epidural or spinal anaesthesia

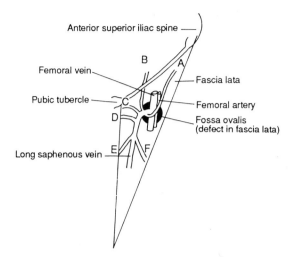

Figure 13.3 The femoral triangle showing the entrance of the long saphenous vein through the fossa ovalis into the femoral vein. The tributaries of the long saphenous vein are labelled as follows: A, superficial circumflex iliac; B, superficial epigastric; C, superficial external pudendal; D, deep external pudendal; E, medial femoral; F, lateral femoral

Q14
A. **True** – For compartment syndrome
B. **True** – For acute renal failure
C. **False** – Alkaline forced diuresis may be required. Myoglobulin precipitates in acid urine
D. **True**
E. **True**

Q15
A. **False** – AAA is the commonest aneurysm
B. **False** – It is usually caused by artherosclerosis
C. **False** – Angiography is not essential
D. **False** – This is true of popliteal aneurysms. The femoral artery is excised or the sac is closed over an inlay graft
E. **True** – Thrombosis and rupture are also recognised complications

Q16
A. **False** – The thrombogenicity potential is lower
B. **False** – Revision is more difficult because of adherence to surrounding tissue
C. **True**
D. **True** – Causing stenosis
E. **False** – They dilate in response to papaverine, which is used to overcome graft spasm

Q17
A. **True**
B. **False** – The activated partial thromboplastin (APTT) is used to monitor heparin anticoagulation. INR is used to monitor warfarin anticoagulation
C. **True**
D. **False** – It has a shorter duration of action
E. **False** – This regimen is suitable for prophylaxis in high-risk patients

Q18
A. **True**
B. **True**
C. **False** – Horner's syndrome is caused by interruption of sympathetic outflow to the head and neck
D. **False** – This drug is a vasodilator (α-blocker)
E. **True**

Q19
A. **True** – Due to cystic accumulation of mucopolysaccharides in the medial layer
B. **False** – They start in the ascending aorta
C. **True**
D. **True** – Due to cardiac tamponade
E. **False** – This condition should be differentiated from MI

Q20
A. **True**
B. **True**
C. **False**
D. **True**
E. **False**

Q21
A. **False** – The knitted Dacron grafts require preclotting
B. **False** – They consist of polyethylene fibres
C. **True**
D. **False** – PTFE grafts are preferred
E. **True** – To reduce porosity and blood loss

Q22
A. **True** – This results from injury to the artery of Adamkiewicz
B. **True** – For example, owing to aortoduodenal fistula
C. **True**
D. **True**
E. **True**

Q23
A. **False** – It is more common in women
B. **True** – Selective venous sampling may be used in diagnosis
C. **True**
D. **False** – Medical management is less desirable than surgery in children
E. **False** – Hypertension may be cured in 90% of such cases

Q24
A. **False** – *Staphylococcus aureus* is usually responsible
B. **True**
C. **False** – *Helicobacter pylori*, which is associated with peptic ulceration and gastric cancer, has not been reported as a cause of graft infection
D. **True**
E. **False** – Radical or limited surgery is often necessary

Q25
A. **False** – These are a trigger factor
B. **True**
C. **False** – This is a trigger factor
D. **True**
E. **True** – Proprietary name Praxilene®

Q26
A. **True**
B. **False** – They expand at 0.4 cm per year
C. **True**
D. **True** – In mycotic aneurysms
E. **False** – The 5 year rupture rate is 75% in this case

Q27
A. **True** – Due to extravasation of sclerosant
B. **False** – This complicates trauma
C. **True**
D. **False** – This is a synonym for mycetoma pedis (chronic fungal infection)
E. **True**

Q28
A. **False** – This is caused by multiple arterial emboli
B. **False** – This is a sign of congenital arteriovenous fistulae. In this sign proximal compression over the artery decreases the swelling and pulse rate
C. **True** – Due to haemosiderin
D. **True**
E. **False** – The pain is typically relieved by elevating the limb (venous claudication)

Q29
A. **True** – Due to impaired venous and lymphatic return
B. **True** – Due to compression of the axillary artery and/or vein
C. **True**
D. **True** – Due to embolic episodes
E. **False**

Q30
A. **False** – Cervical sympathectomy may be performed
B. **True**
C. **False** – Prolapsed intervertebral cervical disc can cause symptoms mimicking TOS
D. **True**
E. **True** – This helps symptoms in 75% of patients if there is no cervical rib

Q31
A. **True**
B. **False** – This shunt drains peritoneal fluid (ascites) into a main vein
C. **True** – In this procedure a dermal flap is buried into swollen tissue
D. **True** – Pulsatile compression devices may be used
E. **False** – This open-palm technique is used for Dupuytren's contracture

Q32
A. **False** – Milroy's disease accounts for less than 10% of cases
B. **True**
C. **False** – This parasite causes secondary lymphoedema
D. **False**
E. **False** – This is a feature of venous hypertension
Note: Primary lymphoedema includes lymphoedema congenita (in infancy), lymph-oedema praecox (in the second and third decades) and lymphoedema tarda (after 30 years). Lymphoedema praecox is the commonest type

Q33
A. **True** – Due to motor neuropathy affecting the small muscles of the foot. The action of the long flexors is unopposed
B. **True** – Due to neuropathy
C. **True**
D. **False** – Autonomic neuropathy is usually present
E. **True** – Due to ischaemia

Q34
A. **False** – Most patients are young men who smoke
B. **True**
C. **False** – The major histological changes occur in the intima. The erythrocyte sedimentation rate is usually normal
D. **True**
E. **True**

Q35
A. **False** – Deep vein thrombosis is the commonest cause
B. **True**
C. **False** – Sclerosants include 3% sodium tetradecyl sulphate (STD) and ethanolamine
D. **False** – They are usually acquired and caused by incompetent valves
E. **True**

Q36
A. **True** – Or cervical block
B. **True**
C. **False** – It is not essential to use a shunt
D. **True**
E. **False** – The acceptable mortality rate should be less than 5%

Q37
A. False
B. True
C. False
D. True
E. True

Q38
A. **False** – This predicts a good healing rate
B. **False** – This predicts a good healing rate
C. **False**
D. **False**
E. **True** – There is no absolute predictor of healing in below-knee amputation

Q39
A. **True** – The nerve should be divided cleanly and allowed to retract to avoid painful neuroma formation
B. **False**
C. **True** – This usually fades with time
D. **True**
E. **True** – This tends to occur in patients with peripheral vascular disease. The use of antibiotics active against gas gangrene organisms reduces its incidence

Q40
A. **False** – This predicts a good healing rate
B. **True**
C. **False**
D. **True**
E. **True**

Q41
A. **False** – Elevation reduces the blood supply
B. **True** – Systemic or topical
C. **True**
D. **True**
E. **False** – These are useful in venous insufficiency

Q42
A. **False** – They are the most common benign tumours of the lymphatics
B. **True** – In this location, they can cause respiratory distress
C. **True** – Also in the axilla or mediastinum
D. **True** – To avoid respiratory distress
E. **False** – These tumours are benign

Q43
A. **False** – Complete occlusion is a contraindication
B. **True** – LSV grafts have a greater patency rate than synthetic grafts such as GORE-TEX®
C. **True**
D. **False**
E. **False** – β-Blockers reduce cardiac output and blood pressure, and therefore should not be used

14. Gastrointestinal Surgery

Q1 **The complications of ulcerative colitis include:**

A. Colonic strictures in 10% of cases
B. Anal fissures
C. Colonic perforation in 25% of hospitalised patients
D. Sclerosing cholangitis in 10% of cases
E. Arthropathy in 1% of cases

Q2 **Gastrointestinal carcinoid tumours:**

A. Most commonly occur in the jejunum
B. May cause appendicitis
C. Are derived from apudomas
D. Have a prognosis that is independent of tumour size
E. Are multicentric in 50% of cases

Q3 **Meckel's diverticulum:**

A. Is caused by failure of the vitellointestinal duct to close at the intestinal end
B. Most commonly presents as diverticulitis
C. May contain pancreatic tissue
D. Excision is recommended only in symptomatic cases
E. Predisposes to small bowel volvulus

Q4 **When performing an appendicectomy through the gridiron incision the surgeon will encounter:**

A. The fibres of the external oblique muscle lying perpendicular to the line of incision
B. The fibres of the internal oblique and transversus abdominis lying almost in a transverse direction
C. Scarpa's fascia deep to the external oblique aponeurosis
D. The trasversalis fascia fused to the peritoneum
E. Numerous communications between the appendicular artery and the ileal arteries

Q5 **With respect to inguinal hernias:**

A. The sac of the direct hernia bulges lateral to the inferior epigastric artery
B. The neck of an indirect hernia lies lateral to the inferior epigastric artery
C. The direct variety is more common in children
D. The direct variety is more common in older men
E. An indirect hernia is more likely to strangulate than a direct hernia

Q6   The following statements about the inguinal canal are true:

A. The medial part of the inferior wall is formed by the lacunar ligament
B. The superior wall is formed by the lowest fibres of the external oblique
C. The posterior wall is reinforced in its lateral third by the conjoint tendon
D. The anterior wall is reinforced in its lateral third by the fibres of origin of the internal oblique
E. The deep inguinal ring lies medial to the inferior epigastric vessels

Q7   In the treatment of Crohn's disease of the small bowel:

A. Corticosteroids are effective in the acute phase
B. Surgical resection of the involved segment has a 5% recurrent rate
C. Aluminium hydroxide may alleviate diarrhoea
D. Surgery is indicated only to deal with complications
E. Bulk-forming drugs are recommended

Q8   Carcinoid syndrome:

A. Occurs only in the presence of liver metastases
B. Diagnosis is made by finding elevated levels of 5-hydroxyindoleacetic acid in urine
C. Due to a bowel primary has a 5 year survival rate of 20%
D. Usually responds to pharmacological treatment
E. Causes mitral valve stenosis

Q9   Adenocarcinoma of the small bowel:

A. Is most commonly located in the ileum
B. Is less common than small bowel lymphoma
C. Is a recognised cause of intussusception
D. Shows metastases in a large number of patients at laparotomy
E. May arise from benign adenomatous polyps

Q10   The following statements about the blood supply of the small and large intestine are true:

A. The upper half of the duodenum is mainly supplied by the inferior pancreatico-duodenal artery
B. The jejunum and ileum are supplied by branches of the superior mesenteric artery
C. The caecum is supplied by the middle colic artery
D. The distal third of the transverse colon is mainly supplied by the ileocolic artery
E. The descending colon is supplied by the inferior mesenteric artery

Q11   When performing a highly selective vagotomy for duodenal ulcer, the surgeon usually:

A. Finds that the anterior vagus gives off the branches to the liver and gall bladder
B. Finds the posterior vagus as a thick cord closely applied to the oesophagus
C. Denervates the parietal area of the stomach
D. Divides the coeliac branch of the posterior vagus
E. Performs pyloroplasty

Q12 Adult pyloric stenosis:

A. Is usually caused by duodenal ulceration
B. May be caused by gastric ulceration
C. Often causes hyperkalaemia
D. Usually causes metabolic acidosis
E. Is often treated with nasogastric tube and omeprazole

Q13 Crohn's disease:

A. Has a mean age of onset of 25 years
B. Is commoner in tropical areas
C. May affect the mouth
D. Spares the bowel mesentery
E. Incidence is decreased by vaccination against measles virus

Q14 Consider the post-contrast computed tomogram of the abdomen shown in Figure 14.1. The following statements are true:

A. N is the main portal vein
B. M is the common bile duct
C. P is the left kidney
D. T is the inferior vena cava
E. This cut lies at the level of the second lumbar vertebra

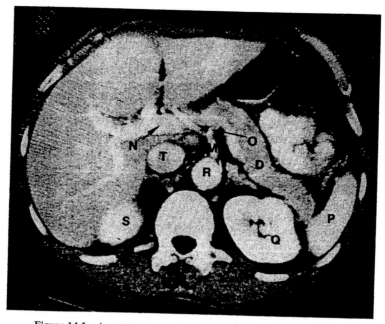

Figure 14.1   A post-contrast computed tomogram of the abdomen

Q15 The following differences help the operating surgeon to distinguish between jejunum and ileum

A. The calibre of the small bowel diminishes from the proximal jejunum to the distal ileum
B. Peyer's patches are more numerous in the ileum than in the jejunum
C. The ileal mesentery is thinner and more translucent than that of the jejunum
D. There is a more marked tendency towards arborisation and anastomosis of vascular arcades in the jejunal mesentery than in the ileal mesentery
E. The lymphatics and lymph nodes are more numerous and larger in the ileal mesentery than in the jejunum

Q16 The rectum:

A. The rectum begins at the level of the third sacral vertebra
B. The rectum has peritoneal covering throughout its length
C. The rectum exhibits three lateral curves: two with convexities towards the left and one with its convexity towards the right
D. Denonvillers' fascia is more developed in the female than in the male
E. The middle and inferior rectal arteries are branches of the inferior mesenteric artery

Q17 The complications of Crohn's disease include:

A. Small bowel strictures
B. Macrocytic anaemia
C. Ileovesical fistula formation
D. Necrobiosis lipoidica diabeticorum (NLD)
E. Localised abscess around the ileum

Q18 The following clinical presentations are more common in right-sided colonic cancers than in left-sided colonic cancers:

A. Bright red rectal bleeding
B. Bowel obstruction
C. Microcytic hypochromic anaemia
D. An abdominal mass
E. Change of bowel habits

Q19 Volvulus of the sigmoid colon:

A. Has an incidence that is decreased by a high-fibre diet
B. Causes asymmetrical distension of the abdomen
C. Is usually diagnosed by plain abdominal radiographs
D. Requires laparotomy in all cases
E. Can be treated conservatively by placing the patient in the knee–elbow position, sigmoidoscopy and gentle passing of a flatus tube

Q20 Portosystemic anastomoses occur:

A. Around the umbilicus
B. In the middle third of the oesophagus
C. In the lower end of the rectum
D. In the bare area of the liver
E. In the appendix

Q21   With respect to the spleen:

A. The splenic artery passes to the spleen through the gastrosplenic ligament
B. The lienorenal ligament contains the tail of the pancreas
C. Most laterally, the spleen is in contact with the phrenicocolic ligament
D. Segmental resection of the spleen is possible owing to its segmental blood supply
E. Spontaneous splenic rupture is a recognised feature of chronic myelocytic leukaemia

Q22   The consequences of resection of the terminal ileum include:

A. Subacute combined degeneration of the spinal cord
B. Diarrhoea
C. Decreased incidence of gallstone formation
D. Pernicious anaemia
E. Peripheral neuropathy

Q23   Ulcerative colitis:

A. Is more common in females than in males
B. Usually presents in the fifth decade
C. Is associated with proctitis in most cases
D. Frequently involves the jejunum
E. Has an increased incidence of colorectal malignancy

Q24   Ischaemic colitis:

A. Most commonly involves the splenic flexure
B. Shows thickening of the involved bowel segment on barium enema
C. May cause colonic strictures
D. Is treated with prednisolone
E. Should be treated with urgent colectomy once diagnosed

Q25   Villous adenoma:

A. Is a recognised cause of hypokalaemia
B. Is commoner in the right colon than in the left colon
C. Secretes 5-hydroxytryptamine (5-HT)
D. May be treated with local excision
E. Has a greater malignant potential than tubular adenoma

Q26   The following results exclude appendicitis as a cause of pain in the right iliac fossa:

A. Microscopic haematuria
B. Normal white cell count
C. Normal ultrasonography
D. Normal levels of C-reactive protein in serum
E. Lack of tenderness on digital rectal examination

Q27   Acute appendicitis:

A. Usually causes a high fever in the early stages
B. Causes central abdominal pain in the early stages
C. May cause microscopic haematuria
D. Is usually caused by obstruction of the appendicular lumen
E. Is commoner in males

Q28   Acute appendicitis:

A. Has a peak incidence in the first decade of life
B. Is the commonest condition requiring emergency surgery
C. Usually causes vomiting, which precedes abdominal pain
D. During pregnancy should be treated conservatively
E. Causes anorexia in most patients

Q29   In complete acute obstruction of the small intestine:

A. Initially there is intermittent colicky pain, which is sharply localised
B. The gas in the distended bowel is mainly methane and hydrogen disulphide produced in the intestine
C. The flux of fluids and electrolytes from the lumen back into the tissue is markedly reduced in the obstructed segment
D. The obstructed segment provides a good environment for bacterial proliferation
E. The intraluminal pressure does not exceed $10\,cmH_2O$

Q30   Motility of the small intestine may be reduced by:

A. Neostigmine
B. Abdominal exploration
C. Morphine
D. Vagotomy
E. Excessive hydroxytryptamine (5-HT) secretion in the carcinoid syndrome

Q31   The following statements about bilirubin and its metabolites are true:

A. Bilirubin is nephrotoxic
B. The conjugation of bilirubin is performed by the β-glucuronidase enzymes
C. The conjugated bilirubin is secreted into the bile by simple diffusion
D. A fraction of urobilinogen is reabsorbed from the intestine and re-excreted through the liver
E. Urobilins are colourless compounds

Q32   The clinical signs of acute appendicitis include:

A. Grey Turner's sign
B. Rovsing's sign
C. Psoas sign
D. Cullen's sign
E. Obturator sign

ie complications of haemorrhoidectomy include:

tenosis
urinary retention
yaemia
laemic shock
E. Flatus incontinence

Q34 Anal fissures:

A. Usually lie posteriorly
B. Located anteriorly are commoner in men
C. Are commonly associated with sentinel tags
D. Are best treated with Lord's procedure
E. Are relatively common in Crohn's disease

Q35 With respect to bile:

A. About 2 litres of bile are secreted into the duodenum daily
B. Most of the bile acids are reabsorbed in the colon
C. Some of the urobilinogen absorbed in the colon is excreted in the urine
D. The solubility of cholesterol in the bile is independent of its relative molar concentration
E. Cholecystokinin–pancreozymin (CCK-PZ) causes bile secretion into the duodenum

Q36 Exocrine pancreatic secretion may be stimulated by:

A. Gastrin
B. Secretin
C. Atropine
D. Cholecystokinin-pancreozymin (CCK-PZ)
E. Vasoactive intestinal polypeptide (VIP)

Q37 The following transmitter substances increase intestinal secretion of water and electrolytes:

A. Noradrenaline
B. VIP (vasoactive intestinal polypeptide)
C. Prostaglandins
D. Dihydroxy bile acids
E. Acetylcholine

Q38 Haemorrhoids:

A. Are the commonest cause of bright red rectal bleeding
B. Represent varicosities of the anal veins
C. Of first degree are treated with injection sclerotherapy
D. Are usually located in the 4, 6 and 11 o'clock positions
E. Commonly cause pruritus ani

Q39 Anal fistulae:

A. Usually arise from infected anal glands
B. Commonly present with pruritus
C. Usually resolve with conservative management
D. Are associated with ulcerative colitis
E. With anterior external openings usually open in the midline of the anus

Q40 In the treatment of anal fistulae:

A. Subcutaneous fistulae are laid open
B. Fistulae lying above the anorectal ring are usually laid open in a one-stage operation
C. A non-absorbable stout ligature has a role in the management of subcutaneous fistulae
D. Faecal incontinence is a recognised complication of treatment
E. A high-fibre diet is the mainstay of conservative management

Q41 Total parenteral nutrition (TPN):

A. Contains protein in the form of hydrolysates of casein
B. Contains albumin
C. Should be enriched with aromatic amino acids in patients with hepatic failure
D. May be complicated by hyperosmolar crisis
E. Contains zinc and copper

Q42 Omeprazole:

A. Is a proton pump inhibitor
B. Is the most effective agent in reflex oesophagitis
C. Can eradicate *Helicobacter pylori*
D. Has been shown to produce carcinoid tumours in rats when used in high doses
E. Is ineffective in the treatment of Zollinger–Ellison syndrome

Q43 A complete rectal prolapse:

A. Is frequently seen in infants
B. Involves all layers of the rectal wall
C. May be complicated by gangrene of the rectum
D. Is commoner in males
E. Is usually treated with transabdominal rectopexy in the fit patient

Q44 The following are recognised treatments of a rectal prolapse:

A. Thiersch wire around the anal orifice
B. Delorme's procedure
C. Lord's operation
D. Laparoscopic rectopexy with a Prolene® mesh
E. Lateral internal sphincterotomy

Q45 Colorectal carcinoma:

A. Associated with liver metastases should not be treated surgically
B. Does not respond to radiotherapy
C. Tumour marker is carcino-embryonic antigen (CEA)
D. Of Dukes' stage C is commonly treated with postoperative 5-fluorouracil
E. Size is the best prognostic indicator

Q46 The following are commoner in Crohn's disease than in ulcerative colitis:

A. Crypt abscesses in the bowel mucosa
B. Pseudopolyps in the bowel lumen
C. The development of carcinoma as a complication
D. Bowel obstruction as a complication
E. Involvement of the submucosa and deeper layers

Q47 Cholesterol gallstones:

A. Are usually multiple, small and hard
B. Do not form in bile that contains a 3% molar concentration of cholesterol
C. Have an incidence that is increased in patients with diabetes mellitus
D. May be visible on a plain abdominal radiograph
E. Commonly develop in long-standing haemolytic anaemias

Q48 The consequences of chronic liver failure include:

A. Hypergammaglobulinaemia
B. Hypoalbuminaemia
C. Encephalopathy
D. Low plasma levels of von Willebrand's factor
E. Hypercholesterolaemia

Q49 In the surgical treatment of colorectal cancer:

A. The distal margin is more important than the proximal margin
B. The mesentery should be excised
C. Liver resection is indicated for metastases involving both liver lobes
D. Normal saline lavage during colectomy reduces the incidence of local recurrence
E. The incidence of blood–bone metastases is reduced by early control of the main artery supplying the tumour during tumour manipulation

Q50 Liver abscess:

A. Is caused by colonic diverticulitis in most cases
B. Can clinically simulate acute cholecystitis
C. Causes jaundice in most cases
D. Usually requires laparotomy for drainage
E. Is treated with ultrasound-guided percutaneous drainage

Q51 Hydatid cyst of the liver:

A. Is commoner among urban subjects
B. Is due to *Echinococcus granulosus*
C. Is a recognised cause of anaphylactic shock
D. Is treated with controlled rupture of the cyst, followed by its removal
E. Rarely ruptures

Q52 In the management of portal hypertension:

A. Portocaval shunting has a 10% operative mortality rate for Child class C
B. Portocaval shunting has a 2% operative mortality rate for Child class A
C. Portocaval shunting stops acute variceal haemorrhage in approximately 95% of cases
D. Frusemide is the diuretic of choice for hepatic ascites
E. A Sengstaken–Blakemore tube controls bleeding in 70% of patients with variceal haemorrhage

Q53 Variceal haemorrhage:

A. Treatment includes laxatives
B. Recurrence is reduced by 90% with endoscopic sclerotherapy
C. Recurrence is not reduced with portosystemic shunting
D. May be treated with somatostatin
E. May precipitate hepatic encephalopathy

Q54 Clinical features supporting the possibility of bowel strangulation include:

A. Leukocytosis
B. High blood pH
C. Pyrexia
D. Localised tenderness
E. Bradycardia (in the early stage)

Q55 Large bowel obstruction:

A. Is most commonly caused by diverticular disease
B. Produces early symptoms including nausea and vomiting
C. Is usually located in the left hemicolon
D. Causes colicky lower abdominal pain
E. Is the commonest indication for Hartmann's operation

Q56 Colonic angiodysplasia:

A. Is commoner in the left hemicolon
B. Is associated with pyoderma gangrenosum
C. Related haemorrhage may respond to peripheral intravenous vasopressin
D. Related bleeding usually resolves spontaneously
E. Increases the risk of colonic carcinoma

Q57 Recognised treatments for bleeding colonic angiodysplasia include:

A. Subtotal colectomy
B. Peripheral intravenous vasopressin
C. Colonoscopic argon laser
D. Peripheral intravenous papaverine
E. Colonoscopic electrocoagulation

Q58 Recognised causes of colovesical fistula include:

A. Radiotherapy to the pelvis
B. Carcinoma of the sigmoid colon
C. Diverticulitis
D. Crohn's disease
E. Irritable bowel syndrome

Q59 In the postoperative period following splenectomy:

A. Subphrenic abscess is the commonest complication
B. Overwhelming sepsis occurs only in children
C. About 80% of septic episodes occur within 2 years
D. Polyvalent pneumococcal vaccine will protect patients from 99% of pneumococci
E. Thrombocytosis does not require treatment

Q60 The indications for total parenteral nutrition (TPN) include:

A. Irritable bowel syndrome
B. Pancreatitis
C. Unresolving motor dysphagia due to cerebrovascular accident
D. Gastrointestinal fistula
E. Prolonged paralytic ileus

Q61 Recognised causes of paralytic ileus include:

A. Diabetic ketoacidosis
B. Retroperitoneal haematoma
C. Thyrotoxicosis
D. Hypokalaemia
E. Acute pancreatitis

Q62 The following are recognised complications of pancreatic fistula:

A. Metabolic alkalosis
B. Haemorrhage
C. Renal failure
D. Septicaemia
E. Malnutrition

Q63 Factors responsible for failure of spontaneous closure of a gastrointestinal fistula include:

A. Distal obstruction
B. Lack of epithelial lining of the fistulous tract
C. Foreign bodies
D. Cancer at the fistula site
E. Use of systemic antibiotics

Q64 Ischaemic colitis:

A. Commonly involves the rectum
B. Is characterised by rectal bleeding followed by abdominal pain
C. Causes thumb printing on barium enema
D. Should be treated surgically once diagnosis is made
E. Is a recognised cause of colonic strictures

Q65 The following are recognised complications of diverticulitis:

A. Colonic stricture
B. Irritable bowel syndrome
C. Colo-uterine fistula
D. Haemorrhage
E. Endotoxic shock

Q66 Diverticular disease of the colon:

A. Often affects the rectum
B. Most commonly affects the sigmoid colon
C. Is characterised by true colonic diverticulae
D. Has an incidence that is reduced by a high-fibre diet
E. Increases the incidence of colonic carcinoma

Q67 Intestinal lymphoma:

A. Is usually Hodgkin's lymphoma
B. Is a recognised complication of coeliac disease
C. Usually presents with anaemia
D. Is mainly treated by surgical resection
E. Has a 5 year survival rate of 20% following treatment

Q68 Pancreatic pseudocyst:

A. Is lined by epithelium
B. Takes approximately 4 weeks to mature
C. May resolve spontaneously
D. Usually presents as an acute abdomen
E. Is usually treated with surgical excision

Q69 Colonoscopy:

A. Is the investigation of choice for positive faecal occult blood tests
B. Screening in patients with a family history of adenomatous familial polyposis (AFP) should commence at the age of 30 years
C. Is better tolerated by the elderly than a barium enema
D. May cause colonic perforation 72 hours after the procedure
E. Induces haemorrhage in 0.1% of patients

Q70 The complications of endoscopic retrograde cholangiopancreatography (ERCP) include:

A. Retroperitoneal duodenal perforation
B. Pancreatic divism
C. Acute pancreatitis
D. Ascending cholangitis
E. Primary biliary cirrhosis

Q71 The complications of splenectomy include:

A. Acute gastric dilatation
B. Pancreatic fistula
C. Gastric perforation 24 hours after surgery
D. Polycythaemia rubra vera
E. Megaloblastic anaemia

Q72 A 30-year-old man presents with acute abdominal pain, systolic blood pressure of 70 mmHg and rigid abdomen. The following statements are true:

A. The initial investigations should include barium enema
B. The white cell count (WCC) and erythrocyte sedimentation rate (ESR) are the most useful diagnostic tests
C. A Foley catheter should be passed (transurethrally)
D. A gastrograffin swallow is contraindicated
E. The absence of free gas under the diaphragm, on erect radiography, excludes the diagnosis of a perforated peptic ulcer

Q73 Recognised causes of air within the biliary tree on a plain abdominal radiograph include:

A. Choledochojejunostomy
B. Gallstones
C. Cholangitis
D. Zollinger–Ellison syndrome
E. Whipple's procedure

Q74 Splenorenal shunt (Warren shunt):

A. Reduces the recurrence rate of variceal haemorrhage
B. Has a higher incidence of encephalopathy than portocaval shunt
C. Maintains excellent hepatic portal perfusion
D. Is performed mainly for Child's class C portal hypertension
E. Selectively decompresses the mesenteric venous system

Q75 Enteral feeding:

A. Is indicated in Crohn's disease involving the entire small intestine
B. Should be administered as bolus feeds
C. Usually provides 1 kcal/ml
D. Is a recognised cause of oesophagitis
E. Is a recognised cause of diarrhoea

Q76 A 70 kg adult normally requires (in 24 hours):

A. 40 g of nitrogen
B. 150 mmol of sodium
C. 2500 kcal
D. 2.5 litres of water
E. 150 mmol of potassium

Q77 The following statements about lasers are true:

A. Thermal injury is independent of the laser medium
B. Lasers used in gastrointestinal surgery are usually Nd-YAG
C. Light can be transmitted along quartz fibres
D. Lasers may cause cataracts
E. Lasers should not be used in the colon in the presence of irradiation proctitis

Q78 Lasers' therapeutic applications include:

A. Bleeding colonic angiodysplasia
B. Haemorrhoidectomy
C. Palliation of malignant dysphagia
D. Perforated peptic ulcers
E. Villous adenoma in a 90-year-old woman

Q79 Acute pancreatitis:

A. Severity correlates with serum amylase levels
B. Raises serum glucose levels
C. Is a recognised cause of pleural effusions
D. Is a recognised cause of carpopedal spasm
E. Associated with eight signs of Ranson's criteria, has a 50% mortality rate

Q80 Pancreatic adenocarcinoma:

A. Is decreasing in incidence
B. Arising at the tail of the pancreas tends to present earlier than that of the head
C. Confined to the head of the pancreas is treated with Whipple's procedure
D. Is multicentric in 5% of cases
E. Has an overall 5 year survival rate of 25%

Q81 Laparoscopic cholecystectomy:

A. Is contraindicated during pregnancy
B. Has a lower incidence of common bile duct injuries than open cholecystectomy
C. May cause pneumothorax
D. Is a contraindication to the use of Nd-YAG lasers owing to the risk of gas explosion
E. May be complicated by incisional hernias

Q82 The clinical features of hepatic failure include:

A. Ascites
B. Gynaecomastia
C. Encephalopathy
D. Pityriasis rosea
E. Haematemesis

Q83 The following are recognised treatments for bleeding oesophageal varices:

A. Injection sclerotherapy with adrenaline
B. Injection sclerotherapy with vasopressin
C. Oesophageal transection
D. Injection sclerotherapy with glycerine mononitrate
E. Portocaval shunt

Q84 Gallstones:

A. Made of pure bilirubin are the commonest variety
B. May cause small bowel obstruction
C. Are associated with adenocarcinoma of the gallbladder
D. Usually dissolve with the use of oral chenodeoxycholic acid
E. Can be diagnosed by ultrasonography with 99.8% accuracy

Q85 Choledochal cysts:

A. Are usually acquired
B. Usually present with intermittent jaundice
C. Should be treated with surgical bypass of the cyst
D. Of type IV may require liver transplantation
E. Of type III spare the intraduodenal part of the common bile duct

Q86 Acute cholecystitis:

A. Frequently raises the serum amylase
B. Diagnosis is confirmed by finding a "hot spot" at the site of the gallbladder in a HIDA scan
C. Is a contraindication to laparoscopic cholecystectomy in the acute stage (within 72 hours)
D. Is always associated with gallstones
E. Is a recognised cause of peritonitis

Q87 Oesophageal carcinoma:

A. May arise from Barrett's oesophagus
B. Has a worse prognosis if the tumour is diploid
C. Can be accurately staged with computed tomography (CT)
D. Has a better prognosis if palliation is achieved with laser rather than endoscopic intubation
E. Develops in the middle third in most cases

Q88 Bleeding peptic ulcers:

A. Have a mortality rate that is reduced by the use of continuous infusion of H_2 antagonists
B. Should be treated surgically if the blood transfusion required exceeds 7 units
C. Have a re-bleeding rate that is significantly reduced by the endoscopic injection of adrenaline
D. Treated by endoscopic injection of adrenaline have an unaffected mortality rate
E. Usually present as an acute abdomen

Q89 The postgastrectomy syndromes include:

A. Alkaline gastritis
B. Afferent loop syndrome
C. Zollinger–Ellison syndrome
D. Dumping syndrome
E. Ménétrier's syndrome

Q90 The following statements are true of gastric carcinoma:

A. The incidence is decreasing
B. The fungate type is the commonest
C. The 5 year survival rate is > 70% if the serosa and regional nodes are not involved
D. Gastric carcinoma has a similar prognosis to gastric lymphoma
E. The prognosis is not improved if radical *en bloc* dissection of regional nodes is performed

Q91 Duodenal ulcers:

A. Usually affect the second part of the duodenum
B. Have a premalignant potential
C. Causing perforation are usually located on the anterior wall of the duodenum
D. Recur in 7% of patients treated with vagotomy and pyloroplasty
E. Usually heal after a 6 week course of H_2 antagonists

Q92 Gastric cancer:

A. Is commoner in the greater curvature than in the lesser curvature
B. Is multifocal in 40% of cases
C. May complicate atrophic gastritis
D. Is associated with *Helicobacter pylori*
E. Is resectable in 70% of all diagnosed cases

Q93 Highly selective vagotomy (for duodenal ulceration):

A. Has a less than 0.5% mortality rate
B. Has a recurrence rate of 25%
C. May be complicated by avascular necrosis of the lesser curve
D. Is commonly complicated by diarrhoea and dumping
E. Should be combined with gastrojejunostomy

Q94 In the treatment of liver metastases from colorectal cancer, 5-fluorouracil:

A. Is the chemotherapeutic agent of choice
B. Is stabilised by folinic acid
C. Is a recognised cause of mucositis
D. Metabolites inhibit the enzyme thymidylate synthetase
E. Is usually given as repeated bolus intravenous injections

Q95 The management of intestinal fistula includes:

A. Total parenteral nutrition
B. Intravenous antimicrobials
C. Resection of intestinal anastomosis
D. Atropine
E. Cisapride

Q96 Gallbladder cancer

A. Is associated with gallstones in 75% of cases
B. Is squamous cell carcinoma in most cases
C. Often presents with abdominal pain
D. Localised to the gallbladder should be treated by laparoscopic cholecystectomy
E. Involving the gallbladder mucosa only has a 5 year survival rate of 60%

Q97 Anal cancer:

A. Is associated with human papilloma virus (HPV) type 16
B. Often presents with anorectal pain and bleeding
C. Histology reveals squamous cell carcinoma (SCC) in 96% of cases
D. Which is localised to the anus should be treated by abdominoperineal (AP) resection of the anorectum
E. Is associated with inguinal lymphadenopathy in about 20% of cases

Answers to Section 14

Q1
A. **True**
B. **True** – Anal fistulae and anorectal abscesses may also occur
C. **False** – This occurs in 4% of hospitalised patients
D. **True**
E. **False** – This occurs in 10% of cases

Q2
A. **False** – The appendix is the commonest site, followed by the ileum
B. **True**
C **True** – Cells of the amine precursor uptake and decarboxylation (APUD) system
D. **False** – The greater the size, the higher the incidence of metastases
E. **False** – Only small bowel carcinoids tend to be multicentric (and only 30%)

Q3
A. **True** – It therefore contains all coats of the intestinal wall
B. **False** – Peptic ulceration with bleeding is the commonest symptomatic presentation
C. **True** – Or gastric mucosa
D. **True**
E. **True** – Around the fibrous band connecting the diverticulum to the umbilicus (when the band is present)

Q4
A. **False** – The external oblique fibres run parallel to the skin incision
B. **True**
C. **False** – Scarpa's fascia is superficial to the external oblique
D. **True**
E. **False** – The appendicular artery has no anastomosis. This explains the vulnerability of the appendix to necrosis and perforation once the artery is blocked

Q5
A. **False** – It bulges medial to the artery
B. **True**
C. **False** – Inguinal hernias in children are usually indirect in nature
D. **True** – Owing to their weaker abdominal muscles
E. **True** – Owing to the narrow orifice at the internal ring

Q6
A. **True**
B. **False** – It is formed by the lowest arching fibres of the internal oblique and transversus abdominis
C. **False** – This reinforcement lies in the medial third
D. **True**
E. **False** – It lies lateral to these vessels

Q7
A. **True**
B. **False** – The recurrence rate is 50%
C. **True** – By binding unabsorbed bile salts
D. **True** – Such as abscesses, fistulae or obstruction
E. **False**

Q8
A. **False** – Extraintestinal carcinoids may cause the syndrome without liver metastases, e.g. bronchial carcinoid
B. **True**
C. **True**
D. **False**
E. **False** – Tricuspid and pulmonary valve disease may occur

Q9
A. **False** – The duodenum and proximal jejunum are the commonest sites
B. **False** – Adenocarcinoma accounts for 40% of small bowel cancers, whereas lymphoma accounts for 20% of cases (carcinoids account for 30%)
C. **True**
D. **True**
E. **True** – In familial polyposis syndromes

Q10
A. **False** – It is supplied by the superior pancreaticoduodenal artery, a branch of the gastroduodenal artery
B. **True** – These branches lie between the two layers of the mesentery
C. **False** – It is supplied by the ileocolic and right colic arteries
D. **False** – This part of the colon is supplied by the superior left colic artery, which is a branch of the inferior mesenteric artery (IMA)
E. **True**

Q11
A. **True**
B. **False** – It is not applied to the oesophagus, but separated from it by about 10 mm
C. **True** – This is the aim of the operation
D. **False** – The surgeon tries to avoid this
E. **False** – This may be performed in truncal vagotomy to aid emptying of the atonic stomach

Q12
A. **True**
B. **True** – Prepyloric ulcers
C. **False** – Hypokalaemia usually ensues
D. **False** – Metabolic alkalosis usually results from loss of H^+ and Cl^- in the vomitus
E. **True** – If this is unsuccessful, surgical treatment is considered

Q13
A. **True**
B. **False** – It is commoner in northern Europe
C. **True** – Or any part of the gastrointestinal tract
D. **False**
E. **False** – Recent studies have suggested an increased incidence in people who have received measles vaccination

Q14
A. **True** – Dividing into left and right branches
B. **False** – M is the coeliac axis arising from the aorta. It gives rise to the splenic artery, O
C. **False** – P is the spleen
D. **True**
E. **False** – It lies higher. The coeliac axis usually arises at the level of the thoraco-lumbar junction
Note: R is the aorta, D is the pancreas, X is the paravertebral muscles, Q is the left kidney and S is the right adrenal gland

Q15
A. **True** – So does the thickness of the muscular wall
B. **True**
C. **False** – The ileal mesentery is thicker
D. **False**
E. **True**

Q16
A. **False**
B. **False** – The inferior third has no peritoneal covering
C. **True**
D. **False** – This fascia is more developed in the male. It must be identified clearly during surgery in that region
E. **False** – The middle rectal artery is a branch of the internal iliac artery and the inferior rectal artery is a branch of the internal pudendal artery

Q17
A. **True** – Due to fibrosis and inflammation
B. **True** – Due to involvement of the terminal ileum or bacterial proliferation in stagnant loops of the small bowel
C. **True**
D. **False** – NLD is a cutaneous feature of diabetes mellitus. Pyoderma gangrenosum may complicate Crohn's disease. It responds to corticosteroids
E. **True**

Q18
A. **False** – This is more common in left-sided lesions
B. **False** – This is more common in left-sided cancers
C. **True**
D. **True**
E. **False** – The narrower lumen and more solid nature of faeces in the left colon contribute to the presentation with change in bowel habits and obstruction

Q19

A. **False** – A high-fibre diet increases the incidence; therefore, volvulus is relatively common in Africa
B. **True** – Signs are maximal on the left side
C. **True**
D. **False** – Surgery is indicated only in the presence of signs of strangulation or if conservative management fails
E. **True** – If there is no sign of strangulation

Q20

A. **True**
B. **False** – Anastomoses are seen at the lower end of the oesophagus
C. **True** – Between the superior rectal veins (portal) and the middle and inferior rectal veins (systemic)
D. **True** – Between the diaphragmatic veins (systemic) and liver veins (portal)
E. **False**

Q21

A. **False** – This lienorenal ligament transmits the splenic blood supply
B. **True** – Therefore the tail can be damaged at splenectomy
C. **True** – The spleen may be damaged when mobilising the splenic flexure to which the ligament is attached
D. **True** – Two segments are found in 80% of subjects
E. **True** – Minor trauma can cause rupture of pathological spleens

Q22

A. **True** – Due to vitamin B12 deficiency
B. **True** – Due to fat malabsorption and bile salt-induced colitis
C. **False** – The incidence is increased owing to bile salt deficiency
D. **False** – Megaloblastic anaemia due to vitamin B12 deficiency may ensue
E. **True** – Due to vitamin B12 deficiency

Q23

A. **True** – 1.5:1
B. **False** – The disease usually presents in the third decade (20–30 years)
C. **True** – Therefore a sigmoidoscopic biopsy may confirm the diagnosis
D. **False** – Backwash ileitis may occur
E. **True** – The risk increases with duration of disease

Q24

A. **True**
B. **True** – In the early stages
C. **True** – In the late stage
D. **False**
E. **False** – The initial treatment is conservative with fluids, blood transfusion, antibiotics and monitoring

Q25
A. **True** – Due to excessive mucus secretion
B. **False** – Most lesions occur in the sigmoid colon and rectum
C. **False** – This is a feature of carcinoid tumours
D. **True** – Colectomy is indicated for invasion, large lesions (> 2 cm) and familial polyposis. Transanal endoscopic microsurgery (TEM) has been recently used in treatment
E. **True** – Malignancy risk for villous adenoma is approximately 40% (compared with 15% for tubular adenoma). Tubulovillous adenoma has an intermediate risk

Q26
A. **False** – This may occur in appendicitis
B. **False** – The white cell count is frequently normal in this condition
C. **False** – This investigation is useful in diagnosing gynaecological causes of pain in the right iliac fossa
D. **False**
E. **False**

Q27
A. **False** – It causes mild pyrexia (37–38°C)
B. **True**
C. **True**
D. **True** – By lymphoid hyperplasia, faecolith or tumour
E. **False** – The sex distribution is equal

Q28
A. **False** – The peak is in the second and third decades. It is rare at the extremes of age
B. **True**
C. **False** – Such a sequence of symptoms casts doubts over the diagnosis
D. **False** – Appendicectomy is indicated
E. **True**

Q29
A. **False** – The pain is autonomic in nature and therefore not sharply localised. It lies across the abdomen at the level of the umbilicus
B. **False** – The gas is mainly swallowed air
C. **True** – Shields demonstrated this in 1965
D. **True**
E. **False** – It may rise as high as 25 cmH$_2$O

Q30
A. **False** – This increases intestinal motility by inhibiting cholinesterase
B. **True** – Postoperative ileus
C. **True** – Opiates cause constipation
D. **True**
E. **False** – 5-HT increases motility, causing colicky abdominal pain and diarrhoea

Q31

A. **True** – This may be the cause of hepatorenal syndrome (renal failure in jaundiced patients)
B. **False** – These bacterial enzymes deconjugate bilirubin in the intestine
C. **False** – It is secreted against a concentration gradient, therefore an active transport system is required
D. **True** – The enterohepatic circulation
E. **False** – Urobilinogens are colourless, whereas urobilins are coloured

Q32

A. **False** – This is a sign of pancreatitis
B. **True** – Pain in the right iliac fossa on palpation of the left iliac fossa
C. **True** – Pain on extension of the right thigh with the patient lying on the left side
D. **False** – This is a sign of acute pancreatitis
E. **True** – Pain on internal rotation of the flexed right thigh

Q33

A. **True** – Mucocutaneous bridges should be left to reduce the incidence of stenosis
B. **True** – Due to pain
C. **True** – This is uncommon
D. **True** – Due to haemorrhage
E. **True** – Due to damage to the internal anal sphincter

Q34

A. **True**
B. **False** – Anterior fissures are commoner in women due to lack of anterior support
C. **True** – In chronic fissures
D. **False** – Lateral internal sphincterotomy is the operation of choice. Conservative management may be successful
E. **True**

Q35

A. **False** – About 500 ml
B. **False** – Most are reabsorbed in the terminal ileum
C. **True**
D. **False** – The solubility decreases as the relative molar concentration increases (see Figure 14.2)
E. **True** – CCK-PZ contracts the gallbladder and relaxes the sphincter of Oddi

Q36

A. **True** – The sequence of the 5-amino acids at the C-terminal end is identical to that of CCK-PZ
B. **True** – Secretin stimulates electrolyte secretion
C. **False** – Anticholinergic agents reduce secretion
D. **True** – It also causes gall bladder contraction
E. **True** – VIP is similar in structure to secretin

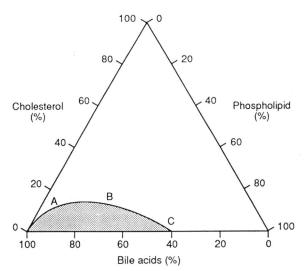

Figure 14.2   Bile samples above the line ABC are supersaturated with cholesterol

Q37
A. **False** – It decreases intestinal secretion
B. **True**
C. **True** – These are thought to contribute to the diarrhoea caused by inflammatory bowel disease and radiation enteritis
D. **True** – They seem to induce colonic secretion
E. **True**

Q38
A. **True**
B. **False** – They are swollen anal cushions
C. **True** – Phenol in oil is usually used
D. **False** – They are usually located in the 3, 7 and 11 o'clock positions
E. **True**

Q39
A. **True**
B. **True**
C. **False** – Fistulae are usually laid open
D. **True** – They are associated with Crohn's disease and tuberculosis
E. **False** – These fistulae open directly into the anus (Goodsall's law)

Q40
A. **True**
B. **False** – The lower track is laid open and a non-absorbable stout ligature is passed through the upper part and left in place for 2–3 weeks. A second operation is required
C. **False** – This procedure has a role in the management of high anal fistulae
D. **True** – Due to possible damage to the anorectal ring (external sphincter)
E. **False**

Q41
A. **False** – It is in the form of crystalline amino acids
B. **False**
C. **False** – These amino acids may precipitate and worsen hepatic encephalopathy. Branched-chain amino acids are recommended
D. **True** – If infusion is given too rapidly
E. **True** – Trace elements should be given daily. Zinc requirements are increased in patients with bowel fistulae

Q42
A. **True** – This reduces gastric acid secretion
B. **True**
C. **False** – Antibiotics are rquired for eradication of *Helicobacter pylori*, e.g. amoxycillin, metronidazole and clarithromycin
D. **True** – Carcinogenicity in humans has not been reported
E. **False**

Q43
A. **False** – Partial prolapse may be seen in children. It is usually self-limiting
B. **True**
C. **True**
D. **False** – It is common in elderly women
E. **True** – Laparoscopic rectopexy and Delorme's procedures are other treatments

Q44
A. **True** – In the unfit patient
B. **True**
C. **False** – This procedure worsens the condition
D. **True**
E. **False** – This may be performed for fissures *in ano*

Q45
A. **False** – Surgery has a role in the local treatment and in the resection of liver metastases
B. **False** – Radiotherapy is frequently used in the pre-operative and postoperative stages
C. **True**
D. **True**
E. **False** – Dukes' stage is the most widely used prognostic indicator

Q46
A. **False** – Crypt abscesses are more conspicuous in ulcerative colitis
B. **False** – These are a striking finding in ulcerative colitis
C. **False** – Carcinoma is less frequent in Crohn's disease
D. **True** – Due to strictures
E. **True** – Crohn's disease is characterised by transmural inflammation

Q47

A. **False** – They are usually solitary, averaging 1.5 cm in diameter and pale brown in colour

B. **False** – See Figure 14.2

C. **True** – Diabetes mellitus is associated with increased cholesterol concentration

D. **True** – A shell of calcium may be deposited on the surface of the stone

E. **False** – Bile pigment stones may complicate chronic haemolytic anaemia

Q48

A. **True** – Less antigen is removed from the portal blood by the diseased liver

B. **True** – Albumin is synthesised in the liver

C. **True** – Ammonia plays an important part in its causation

D. **False** – This factor is synthesised by the vascular endothelium

E. **False** – Cholesterol is synthesised in the liver

Q49

A. **False** – The proximal margin is more important. It should be > 5 cm, whereas the distal margin should be > 2 cm, for adequate excision. The radial margin is also important

B. **True**

C. **False** – Only metastases confined to one lobe are amenable to liver resection

D. **False** – Normal saline is not cytocidal. Sterile water and antiseptic solution have some cytocidal activity

E. **False** – It is common practice to ligate the draining vein early to reduce blood–bone spread, but strong evidence is lacking

Q50

A. **False** – Cholangitis is the commonest cause in the UK

B. **True**

C. **True**

D. **False** – Ultrasound-guided percutaneous drainage and antibiotics are the mainstay of management

E. **True**

Q51

A. **False** – It is commoner in rural areas

B. **True** – Dogs are the definitive host

C. **True** – If rupture occurs

D. **True** – The residual space is then sterilised with a scolicidal solution

E. **False** – This cyst is fragile and commonly ruptures

Q52

A. **False** – The operative mortality rate is 50%

B. **True** – And 10% for class B

C. **True** – With high morbidity and mortality rates

D. **False** – Spironolactone is preferred

E. **False** – The tube controls bleeding in 35%, but bleeding may resume after deflating the tube

Q53
A. **True** – To reduce the incidence of hepatic encephalopathy
B. **False** – Repeated injection reduces recurrence by 50%
C. **False**
D. **True**
E. **True**

Q54
A. **True**
B. **False** – Metabolic acidosis may ensue
C. **True**
D. **True**
E. **False** – Tachycardia is present

Q55
A. **False** – Colonic carcinoma is the commonest cause
B. **False** – These occur late if the ileocaecal valve becomes (or is) incompetent
C. **True** – It is usually located in the sigmoid or descending colon
D. **True**
E. **True**

Q56
A. **False** – It is commoner in the right hemicolon
B. **False** – Pyoderma gangrenosum is associated with inflammatory bowel disease
C. **True**
D. **True** – In most cases
E. **False**

Q57
A. **True**
B. **True** – Vasopressin may also be given via the inferior mesenteric artery
C. **True**
D. **False** – This drug is a vasodilator
E. **True**

Q58
A. **True**
B. **True**
C. **True**
D. **True**
E. **False**

Q59
A. **False** – Atelectasis of the left lower lung is the commonest complication
B. **False** – However, the incidence is higher in children
C. **True**
D. **False** – It protects from approximately 85% of pneumococci
E. **False** – If the platelet count exceeds 750–1000×10^3, antiplatelets (e.g. aspirin) are indicated

Q60
A. **False**
B. **True**
C. **False** – Enteral feeding through a fine-bore nasogastric tube, percutaneous endo-scopic gastrotomy (PEG) or jejunostomy tube is preferred
D. **True**
E. **True**

Q61
A. **True**
B. **True**
C. **False**
D. **True**
E. **True**
Note: Other causes include trauma, septicaemia, major surgery, ganglion blocking drugs, hypomagnesaemia, uraemia and bowel ischaemia

Q62
A. **False** – Pancreatic secretions are rich in bicarbonate, and therefore metabolic acidosis may ensue
B. **True** – The sepsis associated with the fistula may erode a blood vessel
C. **True** – Due to dehydration
D. **True**
E. **True** – TPN may be indicated

Q63
A. **True**
B. **False** – Epithelialisation of the fistulous tract may prevent spontaneous closure
C. **True**
D. **True**
E. **False** – Sepsis may prevent spontaneous closure

Q64
A. **False** – The rectum is usually spared
B. **False** – The bleeding usually follows the pain
C. **True**
D. **False** – The initial management is medical with antibiotics and IV fluids. Surgery is reserved for colonic strictures and colonic perforation
E. **True** – Due to fibrosis of the ischaemic segment

Q65
A. **True**
B. **False**
C. **True** – Colovesical, colovaginal or colo-enteric fistulae may also occur
D. **True**
E. **True**

Q66

A. **False** – The rectum is usually spared
B. **True** – The sigmoid colon has the narrowest lumen
C. **False** – The diverticulae are composed of mucosa and serosa (pseudodiverticulae)
D. **True**
E. **False**

Q67

A. **False** – It is usually non-Hodgkin's, or B cell in origin
B. **True** – This type has a poorer prognosis
C. **False** – It usually presents with subacute small bowel obstruction
D. **True**
E **False** – The 5 year survival rate is > 60%

Q68

A. **False** – The pseudocyst consists of inflammatory products from neighbouring organs
B. **True** – It takes 3–6 weeks to mature
C. **True** – If small in size
D. **False** – The common clinical features include persistent elevation of serum amylase, low-grade fever, a mild leucocytosis and chronic pain
E. **False** – The pseudocyst is usually treated with drainage: percutaneous under ultra-sonographic or computed tomographic guidance, internal (e.g. into the stomach) or external

Q69

A. **True**
B. **False** – It should begin at the age of 20 years
C. **True**
D. **True** – Due to diathermy burns
E. **False** – The incidence is much lower (< 0.03%)

Q70

A. **True**
B. **False** – This is a congenital condition predisposing to pancreatitis
C. **True** – Serum amylase should be measured if abdominal pain develops
D. **True** – Prophylactic antibiotics (e.g. piperacillin) should be given
E. **False** – This is an autoimmune disorder which is relatively common in middle-aged women

Q71

A. **True** – This is treated by passing a nasogastric tube
B. **True** – Due to damage to the pancreatic tail
C. **True** – Due to ischaemia of the greater curve
D. **False**
E. **False** – This may result from vitamin B12 or folate deficiency

Q72
A. **False** – Barium enema should be avoided if viscus perforation is suspected
B. **False** – An erect chest radiograph is the most useful diagnostic test. WCC and ESR are non-specific parameters
C. **True** – To monitor urine output
D. **False** – This may aid the diagnosis of perforated peptic ulcer
E. **False** – Free gas is present in only 85% of perforated peptic ulcer cases

Q73
A. **True**
B. **True**
C. **True** – Due to gas-forming organisms; this is a surgical emergency
D. **False** – This syndrome is characterised by multiple peptic ulcerations due to gastrin-secreting tumours
E. **True** – This includes choledochojejunostomy

Q74
A. **True**
B. **False** – This shunt maintains excellent hepatic portal perfusion, thus decreasing the incidence of encephalopathy
C. **True**
D. **False** – Surgery in this group of patients is associated with excessive morbidity and high mortality rate
E. **False** – It selectively decompresses the splenic venous bed

Q75
A. **False** – Functional small bowel is essential for enteral feeding. TPN is used if the intestine is not functional
B. **False** – It is administered continuously by gravity drip or battery-operated pump
C. **True**
D. **True** – Because of the fine-bore nasogastric tube. This complication is rare
E. **True** – Owing to hyperosmolarity, contamination or bolus feeding

Q76
A. **False** – 10 g of nitrogen
B. **True**
C. **True**
D. **True**
E. **False** – 60 mmol of K^+

Q77
A. **False** – Thermal injury also depends on the wavelength of light used and tissue composition
B. **True**
C. **True** – Therefore they can be used endoscopically
D. **True** – Eyes should be protected with safety glasses
E. **False** – Lasers may be used to treat irradiation proctitis

Q78
A. True
B. True
C. True
D. False
E. True

Q79
A. False – There is no correlation
B. True
C. True
D. True – Due to hypocalcaemia
E. False – The mortality rate approaches 100%

Q80
A. False – The incidence is increasing
B. False – Tumours of the head tend to present earlier because they obstruct the common bile duct and cause jaundice
C. True
D. False – It is multicentric in up to 40%
E. False – The 5 year survival rate is < 5%

Q81
A. True
B. False – The incidence is higher
C. True
D. False – Nd-YAG lasers may be used to dissect the gallbladder from its hepatic bed
E. True – At the portal sites

Q82
A. True – Due to hypoalbuminaemia, hyperaldosteronaemia and portal hypertension
B. True – Due to elevated levels of oestrogens
C. True
D. False – This is a self-limiting skin condition
E. True – Due to variceal haemorrhage

Q83
A. True
B. True
C. True
D. False – Glycerine mononitrate is a vasodilator
E. True

Q84
A. False – Mixed stones containing cholesterol, bilirubin and calcium are the commonest variety
B. True – Gallstone ileus
C. True – 90% of patients with gallbladder carcinoma have gallstones
D. False – Only a minority of stones do
E. False – The accuracy is approximately 92%. Small stones may be missed

Q85

A. **False** – They are congenital
B. **True** – Pain and abdominal mass may also be present
C. **False** – Cysts should be excised to reduce the risk of malignancy
D. **True** – Type IV involves the intrahepatic ducts
E. **False**

Q86

A. **True** – In 13% of patients. The level is lower than that in pancreatitis
B. **False**
C. **False**
D. **False** – Acalculus cholecystitis may complicate trauma, sepsis, burns, etc.
E. **True** – If the gallbladder perforates

Q87

A. **True** – Barrett's oesophagus is a premalignant condition
B. **False** – Diploid tumours have a better prognosis
C. **False** – Magnetic resonance imaging and CT are inaccurate in staging
D. **False** – Survival is the same with the two methods
E. **True**

Q88

A. **False** – H_2 antagonists do not influence the natural history
B. **True**
C. **True** – Adrenaline 1:10 000 should be injected at five sites around the ulcer
D. **False** – The mortality rate is reduced
E. **False** – They usually present as melaena and/or hypovolaemic shock

Q89

A. **True** – This occurs in 25% of cases
B. **True** – Due to intermittent obstruction of the afferent loop of the gastrojejunostomy
C. **False**
D. **True** – Epigastric pain, nausea, palpitations, dizziness and diarrhoea are common symptoms
E. **False**

Q90

A. **True**
B. **False** – This type is less common than the polypoid, ulcerating and diffusely infiltrating types
C. **True**
D. **False** – Gastric lymphoma has a better prognosis (95% is the 5 year survival rate)
E. **False**

Q91

A. **False** – The first part is the commonest site
B. **False** – Duodenal malignancy is rare
C. **True** – Posterior duodenal ulcers may perforate into the lesser sac
D. **True** – Anterectomy and vagotomy procedures have the lowest recurrence rates
E. **True** – Maintenance therapy is often required

Q92
A. **False** – It is commoner in the prepyloric region, antrum and lesser curve
B. **False** – It is multifocal in 12% of cases
C. **True**
D. **True** – There is a recently noted association
E. **False** – The resectability rate is < 50%

Q93
A. **True**
B. **False** – The recurrence rate is 7%
C. **True** – The incidence is < 0.2%
D. **False** – This is rare
E. **False** – This is unnecessary unless there is associated gastric outflow obstruction due to duodenal scarring

Q94
A. **True**
B. **False** – Folinic acid stabilises the active metabolite, 5-fluorodeoxyuridine monophosphate
C. **True** – Leucopenia is another side effect
D. **True**
E. **False** – It is usually given as a continuous venous infusion

Q95
A. **True**
B. **True** – Abscess drainage is also necessary in order to control sepsis
C. **True** – This is often required if conservative management fails
D. **False** – Somatostatin analogues such as octreotide may be used to reduce the fistula's output
E. **False**
Note: It should be remembered that correction of dehydration and electrolyte disturbance is essential in the management of fistulae

Q96
A. **True**
B. **False** – Squamous cell carcinoma accounts for 3% of cases. Adenocarcinoma accounts for 85% of cases
C. **True** – Other symptoms include pruritus, jaundice, weight loss, nausea, vomiting and melaena
D. **False** – Laparoscopic cholecystectomy is associated with portal site metastases and therefore it should be avoided in cancer surgery. Stages I and II can be treated by open simple cholecystectomy
E. **True**

Q97
A. **True** – Other HPV types (18, 31 and 33) have also been implicated
B. **True** – These symptoms are present in 50% of cases
C. **False** – SCC accounts for 80% of cases. Adenocarcinoma and melanoma form the remainder
D. **False** – SCC is primarily treated by radiotherapy and chemotherapy (mitomycin C and 5-fluorouracil)
E. **True** – Inguinal node spread can be treated by radiotherapy or surgery

15. Breast Surgery

Q1   The following are recognised complications of axillary clearance:

A. Arm lymphoedema
B. Winged scapula
C. Costobrachial neuralgia
D. Seroma
E. Subclavian steal syndrome

Q2   Familial breast cancer:

A. Accounts for 20% of all cases of breast cancer
B. *BRCA-1* gene has been cloned
C. Tends to present after the age of 45 years
D. Is a feature of the Li–Fraumeni syndrome
E. Is commonly bilateral

Q3   The current indications for mastectomy include:
A. Centrally located tumours
B. Tumours with extensive intraductal components
C. Paget's disease associated with a breast lump
D. Tumours > 5 cm in size
E. Lobular carcinoma *in situ* (LCIS)

Q4   A 57-year-old woman presented with a 3 cm lump in the upper outer quadrant of the left breast. Mammography did not show any other abnormality. Fine needle aspiration cytology (FNAC) was C5. The following statements are correct.
A. FNAC has a high specificity
B. This patient should be treated with Patey's mastectomy
C. Postoperative radiotherapy reduces local recurrence
D. If the histology shows invasive carcinoma and negative oestrogen receptor status, tamoxifen should not be prescribed
E. Axillary node status is the best single predictor of prognosis

Q5   Ductal carcinoma *in situ* (DCIS) of the breast:

A. Has a well established natural history
B. Usually presents as a palpable breast lump
C. Has a recurrence rate not influenced by postoperative radiotherapy
D. Usually appears as microcalcification on the mammogram
E. Should be treated by adequate excision combined with axillary clearance

Q6   Screening mammography:

A. Is carried out in women aged 50–65 years in the UK
B. Has reduced the breast cancer mortality rate in women over the age of 50 years
C. Should be performed in women aged 30–39 years
D. Has increased the number of DCIS lesions diagnosed
E. Has increased the number of T1 tumours diagnosed

Q7   A 55-year-old woman with a history of breast cancer (20 years ago) presented with skeletal pain. A plain radiograph of the pelvis was arranged (Figure 15.1). This patient:

A. Has widespread skeletal metastases
B. May be treated with tamoxifen
C. May be treated with radiotherapy
D. Should not be treated with formestane
E. Is most likely to have a normal serum alkaline phosphatase level

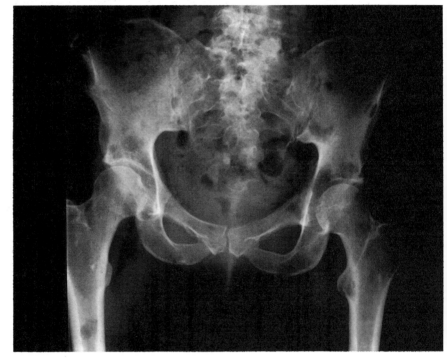

Figure 15.1

Q8   In breast reconstruction:

A. A latissimus dorsi myocutaneous flap is usually used as a free flap
B. The transverse rectus abdominis myocutaneous (TRAM) flap is cosmetically the most superior
C. Becker's prosthesis allows tissue expansion
D. Immediate reconstruction following mastectomy worsens oncologic outcome
E. Full-thickness skin grafts are used for nipple–areola reconstruction

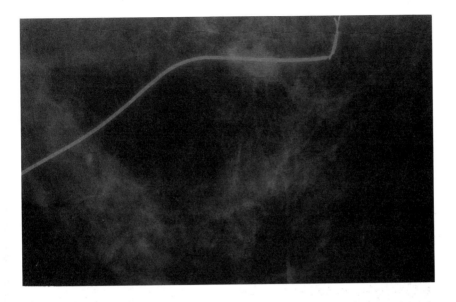

Figure 15.2   Craniocaudal view of the left breast

Q9   Figure 15.2 illustrates a craniocaudal view of the left breast. The following statements are correct:

A. The lesion shown is characteristic of ductal carcinoma *in situ* (DCIS)
B. The lesion is located deep in the breast just lateral to the midline
C. It is not possible to perform fine needle aspiration cytology of this lesion
D. This patient is undergoing wire localisation biopsy because the lesion is suggestive of carcinoma
E. The lesion shown is very likely to be palpable clinically

Q10 Paget's disease of the nipple:

A. Has a prognosis independent of the presence of an underlying breast tumour
B. Does not respond to radiotherapy
C. Is always associated with an underlying breast carcinoma
D. Has a higher incidence in men with Klinefelter's syndrome
E. Is confirmed with an incisional biopsy

Q11 During axillary dissection, the surgeon finds that:

A. The nerve to the latissimus dorsi runs with the vascular pedicle of the subscapularis
B. The long thoracic nerve is closely applied to the chest wall at the posteriomedial aspect of the dissection
C. The pectoralis minor muscle is inserted into the acromion
D. Level III axillary nodes lie lateral to the pectoralis minor muscle
E. The teres major, subscapularis and latissimus dorsi muscles form the posterior axillary wall

Q12 Ductal carcinoma *in situ* (DCIS) of the breast:

A. Presents as a palpable mass in approximately 70% of cases
B. Is associated with positive axillary nodes in 20% of cases
C. Is characterised by microcalcification on the mammogram
D. Treated by mastectomy has a 99% cure rate
E. May become invasive if left untreated

Q13 The following statements about invasive ductal carcinoma (of the breast) are true:

A. It is commonly associated with a family history of breast cancer
B. Its size is the best prognostic indicator
C. Its prognosis correlates well with the number of positive axillary nodes at the time of diagnosis
D. Invasive ductal carcinoma negative for oestrogen receptors never responds to tamoxifen
E. If treated with radical mastectomy, it has better overall survival rates than if treated with breast conservation surgery and radiotherapy

Answers to Section 15

Q1
A. **True**
B. **True** – Due to the long thoracic nerve injury
C. **True** – Due to damage to the costobrachial nerve
D. **True**
E. **False**

Q2
A. **False** – It accounts for 5% of all cases
B. **True** – It has been cloned recently (1994). It has been cloned on 17q21
C. **False** – It tends to present before the age of 45 years
D. **True** – This syndrome is due to a mutation of the *p53* gene
E. **True**

Q3
A. **True**
B. **True**
C. **True**
D. **True**
E. **False** – LCIS is currently regarded as a tumour marker

Q4
A. **True**
B. **False** – Wide local excision combined with axillary clearance is the surgical treatment of choice
C. **True**
D. **False** – Tamoxifen is effective in the absence of oestrogen receptors
E. **True**

Q5
A. **False** – The natural history remains unclear
B. **False** – Lump presentation was common prior to screening mammography, but mammographic microcalcification is now the usual presentation
C. **False** – A recent randomised controlled trial in the USA demonstrated the effectiveness of radiotherapy in DCIS management
D. **True**
E. **False** – The incidence of associated axillary metastases is < 1%

Q6
A. **True** – At 3-yearly intervals. Recent evidence suggests that screening should be performed more frequently and from the age of 40 years
B. **True** – By 30%
C. **False** – There is no evidence of benefit in this age group. Familial breast cancer is an indication for screening mammography before the age of 40 years
D. **True**
E. **True**

Q7

A. **True**
B. **True**
C. **True**
D. **False** – This is an aromatase inhibitor
E. **False** – The serum alkaline phosphatase is usually elevated in such patients

Q8

A. **False** – It is used as a pedicled flap
B. **True** – Particularly if a breast mould and a large volume of tissue are required
C. **True**
D. **False** – There is no evidence for this
E. **True** – Tattooing may increase pigmentation

Q9

A. **False** – DCIS is characterised by microcalcification
B. **True**
C. **False** – The advent of stereotactic technology allows cytology of such impalpable lesions
D. **True**
E. **False** – The need for wire localisation biopsy suggests that the lesion was detected during screening mammography and impalpable clinically

Q10

A. **False** – The presence of an underlying breast tumour indicates a poorer prognosis
B. **False** – Radiotherapy is a recognised treatment
C. **False** – An underlying breast tumour is occasionally absent, thus casting doubt over the traditional theory, which regards Paget's disease as an extension of an underlying breast tumour
D. **True** – It is rare in men. Approximately 50 male cases have been reported
E. **True** – Or scrape cytology

Q11

A. **True**
B. **True** – This nerve supplies the serratus anterior muscle
C. **False** – It is inserted into the coracoid process
D. **False** – These nodes lie medial to the muscle. The muscle insertion into the coracoid process has to be divided to retrieve these muscles
E. **True**

Q12

A. **False** – Approximately 35% of cases of DCIS are palpable at the time of diagnosis
B. **False** – The regional axillary nodes are involved in 1% of cases, therefore axillary dissection is not usually performed for DCIS
C. **True** – This allows early detection by screening mammography
D. **True**
E. **True** – The estimated risk varies from 20% to 60%. Randomised controlled trials are required to determine the true risk

Q13
A. **True**
B. **False** – The number of positive axillary nodes is the best single prognostic indicator
C. **True**
D. **False** – 10% of such tumours respond to tamoxifen
E. **False** – The overall survival rates are similar

16. Endocrine Surgery

Q1   Papillary carcinoma of the thyroid:

A. Is associated with previous neck irradiation
B. Does not metastasise through the blood stream
C. Is usually unifocal
D. Is most common in children and young adults
E. Which has spread to cervical nodes is not curable by surgery

Q2   Following subtotal thyroidectomy for Graves' disease:

A. Exophthalmos regresses
B. Thyroid function tests (TFTs) should be performed within 24 hours after operation
C. The incidence of recurrent laryngeal nerve palsy should be < 1%
D. The serum calcium should be checked within 24 hours
E. The incidence of hypothyroidism is approximately 20%

Q3   A solitary thyroid nodule should be resected (lobectomy) if fine needle aspiration (FNA) cytology shows:

A. Benign follicular cells
B. Atypical cells
C. A cystic lesion which recurs
D. Colloid nodule
E. Chronic lymphocytic thyroiditis

Q4   The following are recognised treatments for Cushing's syndrome:

A. Pituitary radiotherapy
B. Goserelin
C. Trans-sphenoid hypophysectomy
D. Bilateral adrenalectomy
E. Aminoglutethimide

Q5   The clinical features of Cushing's syndrome include:

A. Hyperkalaemia
B. Polycythaemia
C. Pathological fractures
D. Poor wound healing
E. Increased urinary vanillylmandelic acid (VMA)

Q6   The clinical features of phaeochromocytoma include:

A. Postural hypotension
B. Skin pallor
C. Flushing attacks
D. Increased intestinal peristalsis
E. Cardiac dysrhythmias

Q7   Phaeochromocytoma:

A. Arising from the adrenal gland is more likely to be malignant than extra-adrenal tumours
B. Can be diagnosed by measuring serum catecholamines
C. Should be managed pre-operatively with phenoxybenzamine
D. Arising from extra-adrenal tissue is better localised with computed tomography (CT) than with magnetic resonance imaging (MRI)
E. Secretes serotonin

Q8   The clinical features of primary hyperparathyroidism include:

A. Bone cysts
B. Pathological fractures
C. Impaired healing of fractures
D. Tetany
E. Low serum phosphate

Q9   Primary hyperparathyroidism:

A. Is caused by hyperplasia in most cases
B. Is a recognised complication of renal failure
C. Causes subperiosteal bone resorption of the phalanges
D. Should be considered in a patient presenting with constipation and psychosis
E. Causes nephrocalcinosis in 50% of patients

Q10   Thyrotoxicosis:

A. Is caused by Graves' disease in 75% of cases
B. Treated only with carbimazole recurs in 20% of cases within 2 years
C. Is associated with pretibial myxoedema
D. Due to a solitary toxic adenoma, in a 20-year-old woman, should be treated with bilateral subtotal thyroidectomy
E. Recurs in 20% of cases following surgical treatment

Q11   Follicular thyroid carcinoma:

A. Can be excluded if fine needle aspiration cytology shows follicular adenoma
B. Arises from parafollicular cells
C. Commonly presents as cervical lymphadenopathy
D. Should be treated with total thyroidectomy and radioactive iodine
E. Has a 10 year survival rate of 20%

Q12   An asymptomatic diffuse multinodular goitre in a 50-year-old woman should be treated initially with:

A. Subtotal thyroidectomy
B. Observation
C. β-Blockers
D. Thyroxine
E. Propylthiouracil

Q13 With respect to the pituitary gland:

A. The posterior lobe develops from Rathke's pouch
B. The posterior lobe synthesises antidiuretic hormone (ADH)
C. The optic chiasma is separated from the anterior lobe by the diaphragma sella
D. In trans-sphenoidal hypophysectomy the floor of the sella turcica is removed
E. The oculomotor nerve passes in the medial wall of the cavernous sinus lateral to the gland

Q14 Vasopressin (ADH):

A. Is synthesised in the posterior pituitary gland
B. Deficiency leads to a risk of water intoxication
C. Excessive secretion usually results in diabetes insipidus (DI)
D. Primary physiological stimulus is increased plasma osmolarity
E. Acts mainly on the distal convoluted tubules and collecting ducts of the kidney

Q15 The effects of glucocorticoids include:

A. Increased prostaglandin synthesis
B. Decreased number of circulating leucocytes
C. Increased delivery of amino acids to the liver to increase glucose production
D. Suppression of the immune response
E. Potassium reabsorption in the distal renal tubule

Q16 The principal actions of insulin include:

A. Increased lipolysis in adipose tissue
B. Increased ketogenesis in the liver
C. Increased glucose uptake by muscle and adipose tissue
D. Decreased glycogen synthesis
E. Increased protein synthesis

Answers to Section 16

Q1
A. **True**
B. **False** – Although lymph node spread is the commonest mode of metastatic spread, spread via the blood stream is occasionally seen (especially in older patients)
C. **False** – It is usually multifocal
D. **True**
E. **False**

Q2
A. **False**
B. **False** – TFTs may be performed at 6 weeks, because thyroid hormones have a long half-life
C. **True**
D. **True** – Hypoparathyroidism is a recognised complication
E. **True**

Q3
A. **True** – It is impossible to distinguish between follicular adenoma and carcinoma on cytological grounds
B. **True** – This raises the possibility of malignancy
C. **True**
D. **False** – Surgical resection is not mandatory
E. **False** – Surgical resection is not mandatory

Q4
A. **True**
B. **False** – This LHRH analogue is used in the treatment of breast cancer (in pre-menopausal women) and prostatic cancer
C. **True**
D. **True**
E. **True** – This drug inhibits conversion of cholesterol into pregnenolone and inhibits peripheral aromatase, thus causing medical adrenalectomy

Q5
A. **False** – Hypokalaemia is a feature
B. **True**
C. **True** – Due to osteoporosis
D. **True**
E. **False** – This is a feature of phaeochromocytoma

Q6
A. **True**
B. **True**
C. **True**
D. **False** – Parasympathetic stimulation results in increased intestinal peristalsis
E. **True**

Q7
A. **False** – Intra-adrenal phaeochromocytoma is malignant in 12% of cases, whereas extra-adrenal tumours are malignant in 35%
B. **True** – Also urinary VMA
C. **True**
D. **False** – CT is better for adrenal tumours and MRI for extra-adrenal ones
E. **True** – And other hormones

Q8
A. **True**
B. **True** – Due to bone demineralisation
C. **False**
D. **False** – This is usually due to hypocalcaemia
E. **True** – And raised serum calcium

Q9
A. **False** – Parathyroid adenoma is the usual cause
B. **False** – Secondary and tertiary hyperparathyroidism are recognised complications of renal failure
C. **True** – This is a diagnostic feature
D. **True** – Due to hypercalcaemia
E. **False** – Renal calculi occur in 50% of patients, but nephrocalcinosis occurs in only 5%

Q10
A. **True** – Antibodies against thyroid stimulating hormone (TSH) receptors cause diffuse hyperplasia
B. **False** – The recurrence rate is 70%
C. **True**
D. **False** – Total lobectomy is the treatment of choice. Bilateral subtotal thyroidectomy is the treatment of choice for Graves' disease
E. **False** – The recurrence rate is 5%

Q11
A. **False** – It is impossible to distinguish the two pathologies on FNAC grounds alone
B. **False** – Medullary carcinoma arises from parafollicular C cells
C. **False** – Papillary carcinoma metastasises to cervical lymph nodes. Follicular carcinoma spreads via the blood stream to lung and bone
D. **True**
E. **False** – The 10 year survival rate is 40%

Q12
A. **False**
B. **True**
C. **False**
D. **False**
E. **False**

Q13
A. **False** – Rathke's pouch gives rise to the anterior lobe
B. **False** – ADH is synthesised by the hypothalamus. It is secreted by the posterior lobe of the pituitary
C. **True**
D. **True**
E. **False** – The nerve passes in the lateral wall of the sinus

Q14
A. **False** – It is synthesised in the supraoptic nucleus of the hypothalamus and transported to the posterior pituitary via axoplasmic flow
B. **False** – Excessive secretion leads to such a risk as there is impaired water excretion
C. **False** – DI results from deficient secretion or action of the hormone, leading to thirst and polyuria
D. **True**
E. **True**

Q15
A. **False** – Glucocorticoids induce lipocortins, which inhibit phospholipase A2 – thus decreasing the production of prostaglandins and leucotrienes
B. **True**
C. **True**
D. **True**
E. **False** – Glucocorticoids cause Na^+ retention and K^+ excretion

Q16
A. **False** – Lipolysis is decreased
B. **False** – Ketogenesis is decreased
C. **True**
D. **False** – Glycogen synthesis is increased
E. **True** – This is an anabolic effect

17. Paediatric Surgery

Q1   Infantile pyloric stenosis:

A. Is caused by hypertrophy of the longitudinal muscular layer of the pylorus
B. Usually presents in the first week of life
C. Is excluded if the infant passes small frequent stools
D. Can be diagnosed with ultrasound
E. Causes the patient to be frequently hungry and to feed readily

Q2   The biochemical consequences of pyloric stenosis in childhood include:

A. High blood pH
B. Hyperchloraemia
C. Hyperkalaemia
D. Decreased urinary excretion of potassium
E. High serum creatinine

Q3   Intussusception in childhood:

A. Is a recognised complication of Henoch–Schonlein purpura
B. Is most common in infants aged 1–5 months
C. May resolve spontaneously
D. Can be reduced by barium enema in the majority of cases
E. Has, as an early sign, the passage of red-currant-jelly stools

Q4   Inguinal hernias in childhood:

A. Are three times more common in preterm infants than in full-term infants
B. Usually present with pain in the groin
C. May be treated by reinforcement of the posterior wall of the canal
D. Should not be treated surgically until the age of 4 years
E. Are commoner on the right side

Q5   Meconium ileus:

A. Is the neonatal presentation of cystic fibrosis in approximately 45% of cases
B. May be complicated by peritonitis
C. Causes a ground glass appearance on plain abdominal radiographs
D. May be treated with gastrograffin enema
E. Should be treated surgically in all cases

Q6   Hirschsprung's disease:

A. Is caused by the congenital absence of sympathetic ganglial cells in the wall of the colorectum
B. Affects males 10 times more frequently than females
C. Should be suspected if the newborn does not pass meconium in the first 48 hours after birth
D. Involves the rectum in 50% of cases
E. May be treated with the Soave procedure

Q7   Umbilical hernias in childhood:

A. Resolve spontaneously in most cases
B. Should be surgically repaired at the age of 8–12 months
C. Are less common among black children
D. Persisting after the second year of life usually require surgery
E. Are effectively treated with surgical corsets

Q8   Undescended testes:

A. Are due to abnormalities of the Müllerian duct
B. Are frequently dysplastic and atrophic
C. Should be brought down surgically by the age of 2 years
D. May be treated with tamoxifen
E. Are associated with inguinal hernias

Q9   The following are more likely to occur in a patient with undescended testes:

A. Testicular torsion
B. Infertility
C. Testicular trauma
D. Testicular cancer
E. Psychosexual problems

Answers to Section 17

Q1
A. **False** – It is caused by hypertrophy of the circular muscle layer
B. **False** – It presents in the second or third week
C. **False** – This is common
D. **True**
E. **True** – Because the stomach remains empty due to frequent projectile vomiting

Q2
A. **True** – Due to loss of acidic gastric contents
B. **False** – Hypochloraemia usually ensues
C. **True**
D. **False** – The urinary excretion of potassium is increased to reabsorb hydrogen ions
E. **True** – Due to dehydration

Q3
A. **True** – The trigger is an intramural haematoma
B. **False** – It is most common at 6–9 months
C. **True** – However, this is uncommon
D. **True** – This also confirms the diagnosis
E. **False** – This is a late sign indicating bowel ischaemia

Q4
A. **True**
B. **False** – They usually present with a lump in the groin noticed by the parents
C. **False** – Only herniotomy is needed
D. **False** – The hernias should be treated as soon as possible as they tend to strangulate
E. **True** – Because the right testis descends later than the left

Q5
A. **False** – It occurs in 13% of cases
B. **True** – If perforation occurs
C. **True** – Caused by the impacted meconium
D. **True**
E. **False** – Surgery is indicated for perforation and failure of conservative management

Q6
A. **False** – The parasympathetic ganglion cells are usually absent
B. **False** – M:F is 4:1
C. **True**
D. **False** – The rectum is involved in almost all cases, therefore rectal biopsy can confirm the diagnosis
E. **True**

Q7
A.　**True** – Umbilical hernias usually resolve within the first 24 months of life
B.　**False** – Mothers should be reassured, and surgery is recommended if the hernia persists beyond 2 years
C.　**False** – They are commoner among black children
D.　**True**
E.　**False**

Q8
A.　**False** – Undescended testes are associated with abnormalities of the gubernaculum
B.　**True**
C.　**True**
D.　**False** – Human chorionic gonadotrophin (hCG) may be used in treatment
E.　**True**

Q9
A.　**True**
B.　**True**
C.　**True**
D.　**True**
E.　**True**

18. Orthopaedics and Fractures

Q1   In osteoporosis:

A. Bone mass is reduced   T F
B. Matrix formation is increased F
C. Serum calcium is decreased F
D. Plain radiographs are more sensitive than computed tomography (CT) in detecting the disorder F
E. The serum alkaline phosphatase is normal T

Q2   In a healing fracture:

A. Osteoblasts invade the bridging haematoma within 48 hours of injury F
B. The pH of the medium increases gradually T
C. The amount of callus formation is inversely proportional to the mechanical stress at the fracture site F
D. Non-union may be caused by soft-tissue interposition T
E. Bone remodelling is complete within 6 weeks of injury F

Q3   The following bones are particularly vulnerable to avascular necrosis following fracture:

A. Talus T
B. Head of femur T
C. Condyle of mandible F
D. Scaphoid T
E. Third metacarpal bone F

Q4   With respect to the blood supply to the femoral head:

A. The obturator artery supplies the head via a branch that ascends through the femoral neck F
B. The blood supply from the obturator artery is the most important F
C. The medial circumflex femoral artery supplies the head via branches that ascend along the neck deep to the synovial membrane T
D. Extracapsular fractures of the femoral neck severely damage the blood supply to the head F
E. Displaced subcapital fractures of the femoral head seriously damage the blood supply to the head T

Q5   In the knee joint:

A. The anterior half of the medial meniscus is more mobile than the posterior half T
B. The medial meniscus is attached to the superficial fibres of the medial collateral ligament F
C. The suprapatellar bursa almost always communicates with the knee joint T
D. The tibia subluxates posteriorly when the posterior cruciate ligament is torn T
E. The central part of the meniscus is more vascular than its periphery F

144

Q6 **Intertrochanteric fractures of the femur:**

A. Usually cause shortening and internal rotation of the leg
B. Usually disrupt most of the blood supply to the femoral head
C. Are treated with femoral head replacement in most cases
D. Are usually treated with dynamic hip screw (DHS) internal fixation
E. Cause abduction of the leg

Q7 **The complications of tibial fractures include:**

A. Fat embolus
B. Tibial nerve damage
C. Delayed union
D. Compartment syndrome
E. Leg shortening

Q8 **Hip dislocation:**

A. Is usually anterior
B. May cause sciatic nerve injury
C. Is commonly associated with a fracture of the posterior acetabular rim
D. May cause soft-tissue injury within the pelvis
E. Is usually anterior in motorcyclists sustaining a sudden deceleration accident

Q9 **In the wrist, the following structures are found to lie superficial to the flexor retinaculum:**

A. The ulnar nerve
B. The ulnar artery
C. The median nerve
D. The palmar cutaneous branch of the ulnar nerve
E. The flexor digitorum superficialis

Q10 **In the humerus:**

A. The surgical neck lies proximal to the greater and lesser tuberosities
B. The deltoid tuberosity lies halfway down the lateral aspect of the shaft
C. The bicipital groove accommodates the radial nerve
D. The coronoid fossa accommodates the radial head when the elbow is flexed
E. The lateral lip of the bicipital groove receives the insertion of pectoralis major

Q11 **The radial nerve:**

A. Derives its fibres from segments C5–8 and T1
B. Gives off a muscular branch to the biceps
C. Gives off sensory branches to the dorsal aspects of the radial half of the hand
D. Accompanies the profunda artery along its descent in the arm
E. Supplies the triceps

Q12 Mid-shaft femoral fractures:

A. Usually cause the proximal fragment to become extended
B. Usually cause the proximal fragment to become adducted
C. Usually cause the distal fragment to become abducted
D. Rarely cause sciatic nerve damage
E. Commonly cause significant blood loss due to profunda femoris vessel damage

Q13 Intracapsular fractures of the upper end of the femur:

A. Are more likely to be complicated by avascular necrosis of the femoral head than extracapsular fractures
B. Usually occur in post-menopausal women
C. Usually cause shortening and internal rotation of the leg
D. Can be treated conservatively
E. Commonly require femoral head replacement

Q14 In hand infections:

A. *Staphylococcus alba* is the commonest cause
B. Flexor tendon rupture is a recognised complication
C. Paronychial abscess is effectively treated with flucloxacillin
D. Palmar space abscess should be surgically drained
E. Primary suturing should never be performed following surgical drainage of tendon sheath abscesses

Q15 Supracondylar fractures of the humerus:

A. Usually result from direct violence
B. Frequently damage the brachial artery
C. Are usually reduced by traction on the distal fragment, followed by flexion at the elbow
D. Usually occur in children
E. Often cause ulnar nerve injury

Q16 Colles' fracture:

A. Causes the distal fragment to deviate to the ulnar side
B. Typically causes "dinner fork" deformity
C. Is a recognised cause of carpal tunnel syndrome
D. Is reduced by traction, extension and radial deviation
E. Should be reduced and the plaster should be completed immediately

Q17 The complications of pelvic fractures include:

A. Rupture of the puboprostatic ligament
B. Extraperitoneal urinary extravasation
C. Rectal perforation
D. Tearing of the prostate from the membranous urethra
E. Rupture of the internal iliac artery

Q18 The clinical features of a lumbar disc prolapse affecting root S1 may include:

A. Paraesthesia on the medial aspect of the foot
B. A positive femoral stretch
C. Weakness and wasting of the dorsiflexors of the foot
D. Limitation of straight leg raising
E. Impaired knee jerk

Q19 The lateral ligament of the knee:

A. Includes the biceps femoris
B. Is attached to the patella
C. Is tested by applying a valgus strain on the knee
D. Should be treated with crepe bandages and crutches if the injury is associated with instability
E. Injury is frequently associated with posterior tibial nerve palsy

Q20 In fractures of the lateral tibial table:

A. Severe varus stress injury is usually responsible
B. The cruciates may be torn
C. The common peroneal nerve is commonly damaged
D. Associated with 20 mm depression, conservative treatment with skin traction is indicated
E. Open reduction and internal fixation is indicated for fractures depressed by 15 mm

Q21 Avascular necrosis of the femoral head:

A. Commonly complicates intertrochanteric femoral fractures
B. May be caused by internal fixation devices
C. May cause radiographic changes to appear 2 years after fracture
D. May be treated with corticosteroids
E. Is characterised by reduced density of the femoral head on plain radiographs

Q22 In ankle fractures, the indications for open reduction and internal fixation include:

A. Stable fracture of the lateral malleolus
B. Displaced fracture of the medial malleolus
C. Isolated fracture of the posterior malleolus
D. Trimalleolar fracture
E. Bimalleolar fracture

Q23 In ankle dislocations (without a fracture):

A. The medial ligament is ruptured
B. The lateral ligaments are ruptured
C. Avascular necrosis of the talus is a recognised complication
D. The dislocation must be treated with open reduction and surgical repair of ligaments
E. Closed reduction and adhesive strapping is adequate in most cases

Q24 Carpal tunnel syndrome:

A. May cause pain in the forearm
B. Spares the abductor pollicis brevis
C. May be caused by a cervical rib
D. Can be treated with endoscopic division of the flexor retinaculum
E. Diagnosis can be confirmed with the use of electrophysiological tests

Q25 The causes of carpal tunnel sydrome include:

A. Hypothyroidism
B. Rheumatoid arthritis
C. Neuritis of the median nerve
D. Cervical spondylitis
E. Acromegaly

Q26 Osteosarcoma:

A. Patients are aged 10–20 years in 60% of cases
B. Most commonly involves the proximal femur
C. Is best treated with a combination of chemotherapy, radiotherapy and surgical resection
D. Is better outlined by MRI than by CT
E. 5 year survival rate is about 15%

Q27 Techniques known to reduce mechanical loosening of total hip replacement include:

A. Laminar airflow ventilation in the operating rooms
B. Peri-operative corticosteroids
C. Use of a dry operative field
D. Avoidance of cement introduction under pressure
E. Cement restrictors

Q28 Fractures of the patella:

A. Caused by knee flexion are usually comminuted
B. Predispose to osteoarthritis of the patellofemoral joint
C. Are frequently associated with haemarthrosis
D. Should be treated with excision of the patella if comminuted
E. Are frequently treated conservatively with a plaster cylinder

Q29 Rheumatoid arthritis:

A. Usually starts proximally and gradually extends to distal joints
B. Affects females 10 times more commonly than males
C. Clinical features include Heberden's nodes
D. May be treated with penicillamine
E. Is a recognised cause of atlanto-axial dislocation of the cervical spine during anaesthesia

Q30 Osteoarthritis:

A. Causes the joint capsule to become thick and fibrosed
B. Symptoms are worst in the morning
C. Is characterised by osteophytes
D. Is the commonest indication for total hip replacement
E. May be treated with gold salts

Q31 Dupuytren's contracture of the hand:

A. Is associated with liver disease
B. Has equal sex distribution
C. May be caused by allopurinol
D. Most commonly involves the right little finger
E. Is best treated with surgical excision of the fibrotic band

Q32 Slipped femoral epiphysis:

A. Has a peak incidence between 5 and 10 years of age
B. Is often bilateral
C. Is a recognised cause of avascular necrosis of the femoral head
D. Is best diagnosed on an anteroposterior radiograph of the hip joint
E. Should be treated with surgical fixation to prevent further slipping

Q33 Perthes disease:

A. Is avascular necrosis of the femoral head
B. Has a peak incidence between 10 and 20 years of age
C. Is diagnosed with the Ortolani test
D. Should be treated surgically
E. May be treated by long leg cast with the legs held in abduction and internal rotation

Q34 Osteomyelitis in childhood:

A. Is usually haematogenous in origin
B. Is most commonly caused by *Staphylococcus aureus*
C. Usually becomes apparent on plain radiographs 3 days after onset
D. Should be treated urgently with surgical debridement
E. Is ruled out if bone scan is negative

Q35 Anterior shoulder dislocation:

A. Most commonly occurs in epileptics
B. Is a recognised cause of deltoid muscle paralysis
C. Is usually subcoracoid
D. Usually presents with the arm in the adduction position
E. Can be reduced using Kocher's manoeuvre

150

Q36 Following successful closed reduction of fractured tibia and fibula, the plaster cast:

A. Extends from the knee joint to the base of the toes
B. Wedging allows adjustment of minor angulation
C. Should hold the knee joint in full extension
D. Can be changed to a patellar tendon-bearing plaster at 8 weeks
E. Should hold the foot at a right angle

Q37 In the management of fractured tibia and fibula:

A. Rigid compression plating allows faster healing of the fracture
B. Intramedullary nailing is recommended in open fractures
C. Fasciotomy should be performed for compartment syndrome
D. Physiotherapy is of no value
E. Broad spectrum antibiotics are recommended in open fractures

Q38 Paget's disease of the bone:

A. Is commoner in Anglo-Saxon populations than in Africans
B. Is usually associated with hypercalcaemia
C. Is a recognised cause of cardiac failure
D. Increases the risk of osteosarcoma by 5 times
E. May be treated with calcitonin

Answers to Section 18

Q1

A. **True**

B. **False** – This is true of osteomalacia and rickets

C. **False** – Serum calcium is usually normal or slightly increased

D. **False** – CT of the dorsal vertebrae is more sensitive

E. **True** – This enzyme is elevated in osteomalacia

Q2

A. **False** – Fibroblasts and capillaries invade in the initial period

B. **True** – It is acidic initially, then becomes more alkaline

C. **False** – It is directly proportional to stress

D. **True** – Impaired blood supply and inadequate fixation also impair fracture healing

E. **False** – Remodelling takes much longer. Osteoclasts play an important role

Q3

A. **True**

B. **True**

C. **False**

D. **True**

E. **False**

Note: The blood supply comes from distal to proximal in the talus, scaphoid and head of the femur, predisposing them to avascular necrosis

Q4

A. **False** – This branch reaches the head along the ligament of the head

B. **False** – It is less important that the other two routes of blood supply: the retinacular vessels travelling in the posterior capsule and the medullary vessels in the femoral neck

C. **True**

D. **False**

E. **True**

Q5

A. **True** – The posterior half is firmly attached to the deep and oblique portions of the tibial collateral ligament

B. **False** – It is attached to the deep and oblique positions

C. **True**

D. **True**

E. **False** – The central part is avascular. This implies that only peripheral lesions can be repaired

Q6

A. **False** – They cause shortening and external rotation
B. **False** – Most of the blood supply to the head is via the capsular vessels, which usually remain undisturbed
C. **False** – DHS internal fixation is the commonest method
D. **True** – Intracapsular fractures are more likely to cause severe damage to the blood supply of the femoral head and avascular necrosis of the head. Therefore hemi-arthroplasty is more frequently performed for intracapsular fractures and DHS fixation is usually sufficient for extracapsular fractures
E. **False** – The leg may become adducted owing to the unopposed action of the adductors

Q7

A. **True**
B. **True**
C. **True**
D. **True**
E. **True**

Q8

A. **False** – It is usually posterior
B. **True** – In posterior dislocation
C. **True**
D. **True** – In central dislocation, which is usually associated with acetabular fracture (protrusio)
E. **False** – It is usually posterior

Q9

A. **True**
B. **True**
C. **False** – This lies deep to the flexor retinaculum
D. **True**
E. **False** – This lies deep to the flexor retinaculum

Q10

A. **False** – The surgical neck lies distal to the tuberosities, whereas the anatomical neck lies immediately below the head
B. **True**
C. **False** – The spiral groove behind and below the deltoid tuberosity accommodates this nerve
D. **False** – It accommodates the coronoid process of the ulna during elbow flexion
E. **True**

Q11

A. **True**
B. **False** – The biceps is supplied by the musculocutaneous nerve
C. **True**
D. **True**
E. **True**

Q12
A. **False** – The unopposed action of hip flexors causes proximal fragment flexion
B. **False** – The proximal fragment becomes abducted (and externally rotated) due to the action of the gluteus muscles, which are inserted into the greater trochanter
C. **False** – The distal fragment becomes adducted
D. **True**
E. **True**

Q13
A. **True** – Due to disruption of the blood supply to the femoral head
B. **True**
C. **False** – The leg is usually shortened and externally rotated
D. **True** – Undisplaced impacted fractures are occasionally treated conservatively
E. **True**

Q14
A. **False** – *Streptococcus* and *Staphylococcus aureus* are usually responsible
B. **True** – Infection may occur along the synovial sheath of a tendon, causing sloughing of the tendon
C. **False** – Surgical drainage is necessary
D. **True**
E. **False** – Primary suturing is sometimes possible

Q15
A. **False** – They usually result from a fall on the outstretched hand
B. **True** – This may lead to ischaemic contractures of forearm muscles
C. **True**
D. **True**
E. **False**

Q16
A. **False** – The distal fragment deviates radially
B. **True**
C. **True**
D. **False** – It is reduced by traction (to overcome impaction), flexion (to overcome dorsal angulation) and ulnar deviation (to overcome radial deviation)
E. **False** – A radiograph should be taken at 6 days once oedema has settled. The plaster is then completed if the position is satisfactory

Q17
A. **True**
B. **True**
C. **True**
D. **True**
E. **True** – Causing hypovolaemic shock

Q18
A. **False** – The lateral aspect is affected
B. **False**
C. **False** – The plantar flexors are weak and wasted
D. **True**
E. **False** – The ankle jerk is impaired

Q19
A. **True** – And the fascia lata
B. **True** – And the fibula and tibia
C. **False** – It is tested by applying a varus strain
D. **False** – Operative repair is indicated
E. **False** – The common peroneal nerve may be damaged, causing footdrop

Q20
A. **False** – Valgus strain is the usual cause
B. **True**
C. **False** – This is a feature of medial tibial table fractures
D. **False** – If the depression is < 10 mm without associated ligament injury, conservative management is indicated with skin traction (3.5 kg) for about 5 weeks
E. **True**

Q21
A. **False** – It frequently complicates displaced intracapsular fractures
B. **True** – This disrupts blood supply to the femoral head
C. **True**
D. **False** – Corticosteroids may cause avascular necrosis
E. **False** – The density is increased and sphericity is lost

Q22
A. **False** – This is treated conservatively with adhesive strapping or below-knee plaster
B. **True**
C. **True** – Particularly if the fragment is large
D. **True**
E. **True**

Q23
A. **True**
B. **True**
C. **True**
D. **False** – These dislocations are usually treated with closed reduction and plaster fixation for several weeks
E. **False** – Plaster fixation after closed reduction is necessary

Q24
A. **True**
B. **False** – This muscle is innervated by the median nerve
C. **False** – Cervical rib is part of the differential diagnosis
D. **True** – Using a two-portal technique
E. **True**

Q25
A. **True**
B. **True**
C. **False**
D. **False**
E. **True** – Other causes include drugs, pregnancy, Colles' fracture, diabetes mellitus, shoulder immobilisation and amyloidosis

Q26
A. **True**
B. **False** – The distal femur or proximal tibia is most commonly affected
C. **True**
D. **False** – CT is more useful for bony lesions, whereas MRI is more useful for soft tissue lesions
E. **True**

Q27
A. **False** – This may reduce the incidence of infection
B. **False**
C. **True**
D. **False** – Cement should be introduced under pressure to reduce the incidence of mechanical loosening
E. **True**

Q28
A. **False** – Indirect injuries usually cause transverse fractures whereas direct trauma is more likely to cause comminuted fractures
B. **True**
C. **True** – This can be aspirated
D. **False** – Excision is indicated only in very severe cases. It should be avoided when possible
E. **True**

Q29
A. **False** – It usually starts distally and spreads proximally
B. **False** – F:M = 3:1
C. **False** – This is a feature of inherited osteoarthritis
D. **True** – This is a second-line treatment after NSAIDs
E. **True** – Pre-operative cervical spine radiographs are helpful

Q30
A. **True**
B. **False** – This is a feature of rheumatoid arthritis
C. **True**
D. **True**
E. **False** – This is a second-line treatment for rheumatoid arthritis

Q31
A. **True** – Alcoholism, Peyronie's disease, diabetes mellitus, a positive family history and phenytoin therapy are recognised associations
B. **False** – M:F = 10:1
C. **False** – Allopurinol may cause resolution of contracture
D. **True**
E. **True**

Q32
A. **False** – The peak is at 10–20 years
B. **True** – In approximately 20% of cases
C. **True** – Due to disruption of the blood supply
D. **False** – A lateral film is more useful
E. **True**

Q33
A. **True**
B. **False** – The peak is at 5–10 years
C. **False** – This is used to diagnose congenital hip dislocation
D. **False** – Surgical procedures have been developed to keep the femoral head in the acetabulum
E. **True**

Q34
A. **True** – The source may be a boil, urinary tract infection, tonsillitis, etc.
B. **True** – And *Streptococcus pyogenes*
C. **False** – 14–21 days are required for subperiosteal new bone formation
D. **False** – Intravenous antibiotics are the mainstay of management
E. **False**

Q35
A. **False** – Posterior shoulder dislocation is relatively common in epileptics
B. **True** – Due to axillary nerve palsy
C. **True**
D. **False** – The arm is usually in the abduction position (30°) and there is flattening of the shoulder contour
E. **True** – Or the hippocratic method

Q36
A. **False** – It extends from the groin to the base of the toes
B. **True**
C. **False** – It should hold it at a few degrees of flexion
D. **True**
E. **True**

Q37
A. **False** – Fracture healing requires longer in this form of internal fixation
B. **False** – There is a risk of infection. External metal fixation is often used in open fractures
C. **True**
D. **False**
E. **True**

Q38
A. **True** – The incidence increases with age
B. **False** – Serum calcium and phosphate are usually normal. Serum alkaline phosphatase is usually raised
C. **True** – It causes high-output failure
D. **False** – The risk is increased by 30 times. The risk is 10% after 10 years of disease. The disease may cause pathological fractures
E. **True** – This helps bone pain

19. Urology and Renal Transplantation

Q1   Varicocele:

A. Affects approximately 15% of young men
B. Causes Bow sign
C. May be treated with sclerotherapy
D. Is usually treated surgically through a scrotal approach
E. Increases the incidence of testicular cancer

Q2   Renal calculi:

A. Are radiopaque in 90% of cases
B. Of the oxalate variety tend to precipitate in alkaline urine
C. Up to 0.5 cm in size can be managed conservatively
D. Causing acute pyelonephritis should be treated with urgent extracorporeal shockwave lithotripsy (ESWL)
E. In the distal ureter can be removed with a Dormia basket

Q3   In the management of renal calculi:

A. Non-steroidal anti-inflammatory drugs are the analgesics of choice
B. Intravenous urography is the investigation of choice
C. Harder stones are fragmented more easily with ESWL
D. Percutaneous nephrolithotomy (PCNL) is contraindicated in the presence of acute pyelonephritis
E. Ureteroscopy is used in the treatment of ureteric calculi

Q4   Maldescended testis:

A. Occurs in 5% of boys
B. Is commoner on the left side
C. May be treated with human chorionic gonadotrophin (hCG)
D. Malignancy risk is halved with orchidopexy
E. Should be placed in the scrotum at the age of 4 years

Q5   Hydrocele:

A. In the newborn is frequently associated with an inguinal hernia
B. In the newborn should be treated within 6 months
C. Is a recognised cause of testicular atrophy
D. Is a recognised complication of the nephrotic syndrome
E. May be treated with Lord's procedure

Q6   Testicular teratoma:

A. Has a peak incidence 10 years earlier than that of seminoma
B. Diagnosis is usually confirmed with needle biopsy
C. Prognosis is significantly improved with chemotherapy
D. Management includes trans-scrotal orchidectomy
E. Management includes irradiation of para-aortic lymph nodes

Q7   Malignant testicular teratoma:

A. Usually presents with testicular pain
B. Is a radiosensitive tumour
C. May cause a positive pregnancy test
D. Is less likely to metastasise via the blood stream than seminoma
E. Of the trophoblastic variety has the best prognosis

Q8   The kidney:

A. Has a segmental blood supply with profuse anastomoses
B. Is derived embryologically from the mesonephros
C. Tubular function can be assessed by the response to acid load
D. Pelvis peristaltic activity needs a nerve supply
E. Is usually approached surgically through the bed of the 12th rib

Q9   The left ureter:

A. Remains attached to the undersurface of the peritoneum when the peritoneum is reflected
B. Is crossed anteriorly by the left genitofemoral nerve
C. Crosses anterior to the left testicular artery and vein
D. Passes anterior to the fossa intersigmoidea
E. Receives its blood supply from the lateral side of the pelvis

Q10   The principal pathological features of acute kidney allograft rejection include:

A. Thrombosis and fibrinoid necrosis of the medium-sized renal arteries
B. Acellular glomeruli
C. Invasion of tubules by lymphocytes
D. More damage to the medulla than to the cortex
E. Widening of the subendothelial space of the glomerular basement membrane (GBM)

Q11   The bladder:

A. Is separated from the rectum by Denonvilliers' fascia
B. Receives its main blood supply through the inferior vesical artery
C. Pain afferents conducted in sympathetic nerves may reach level T6 in the spinal cord
D. Internal sphincter contracts in response to parasympathetic stimulation
E. Detrusor muscle fibres are arranged in inner circular and outer longitudinal layers

Q12   Irrigating the bladder with glycine solution when performing transurethral resection of the prostate (TURP) may lead to:

A. Increased total body sodium
B. Increased osmolality of the plasma
C. Hyponatraemia
D. Cerebral oedema
E. Hypertension and bradycardia

Q13 ^{99m}Tc DTPA-renogram:

A. Is helpful in the assessment of renal transplant function
B. In a patient with obstructive uropathy is characterised by no rise during phase 1
C. Helps to determine the presence or absence of vesicoureteric reflux
D. Shows hypervascular blush in simple renal cysts
E. Aids the diagnosis of space-occupying lesions

Q14 Recognised causes of haematuria include:

A. Porphyria
B. Papillary necrosis
C. Phenindione
D. Renal tuberculosis
E. Renal infarction

Q15 In intravenous urography (IVU):

A. Free ionic iodine is usually used as a contrast medium
B. The nephrogram may persist up to 24 hours in a healthy subject
C. It is possible to measure "residual urine" accurately
D. The ureters are seen to lie on the tips of the transverse process of the lumbar vertebrae
E. Cardiac arrest is a recognised complication

Q16 In cadaveric kidney transplantation:

A. CD4 and CD8 cells mediate the acute rejection reaction
B. DRw6-negative grafts do better than DRw6-positive ones
C. Multiple blood transfusions prior to grafting increase graft rejection
D. The 5-year survival rate of the transplanted kidney is better for one DR mismatch than for two DR mismatches
E. Cyclosporin A is a useful antirejection therapy

Q17 With regard to human leucocyte antigens (HLAs):

A. The genes are located on the short arm of chromosome 6
B. Class II HLAs are controlled by A, B and C loci
C. Compatibility is more crucial to graft survival than ABO blood group matching
D. Matching at the A and C loci has the greatest influence on graft survival
E. HLAs can be identified by incubating donor lymphocytes with HLA typing sera

Q18 Rupture of the urinary bladder:

A. Is a recognised cause of strangury
B. Is due to trauma in most cases
C. Should be treated with transurethral catheterisation followed by surgical repair
D. Is treated conservatively in most cases
E. Investigations include intravenous urography

160

Q19 Wilms' tumour:

A. Is bilateral in about 10% of cases   T
B. Classically presents with haematuria as an early symptom
C. Is staged as IV if it is bilateral
D. Must be treated with radiotherapy if it is stage 1
E. Is now treated with a 5 day course of cisplatin followed by surgical removal

F

Q20 The following are recognised manifestations of renal adenocarcinoma:

A. Hypercalcaemia
B. Anaemia
C. Finger clubbing
D. Leucocytosis
E. Polycythaemia rubra vera

Q21 The contraindications to extracorporeal shockwave lithotripsy (ESWL) include:

A. Haemorrhagic diathesis
B. A 2 cm ureteric calculus above the iliac crest
C. Distal ureteric obstruction
D. Acute pyelonephritis
E. Pregnancy

Q22 The following are true of renal transplantation:

A. The left kidney is usually placed in the left iliac fossa
B. The renal vein is anastomosed end-to-side to the common iliac vein
C. The renal artery is usually anastomosed end-to-side to the external iliac artery
D. Acute rejection of the graft may be seen during the operation after the vascular clamps are released
E. When the ureter is anastomosed to the bladder, it is possible to establish a reflux-preventing procedure

Q23 Acute pyelonephritis:

A. Is usually caused by haematogenous spread of bacteria   F
B. Gives rise to a palpable kidney in most cases   F
C. Gives rise to pyuria in most cases   T
D. Is more likely to produce renal scarring in children than in adults   T
E. Associated with obstructive uropathy often fails to respond to antimicrobial therapy   T

Q24 Recognised complications of percutaneous nephrolithotomy (PCNL) include:

A. Ureteric obstruction
B. Arteriovenous fistula   T
C. Perforation of the renal pelvis
D. Pyelovenous reflux of irrigating fluid
E. Spastic bladder

Q25 The contraindications for PCNL include:

A. Staghorn calculi
B. Acute hydronephrosis due to a calculus
C. Impacted stone in the upper ureter
D. 2 cm renal stone in pregnant women
E. A staghorn calculus in a patient with an INR of 3.0

Q26 In the management of bladder cancer:

A. Carcinoma *in situ* (Tis) may respond to intravesical instillation of BCG
B. T1 tumours should be treated with transurethral resection
C. Intravesical chemotherapy has failed to reduce the recurrence rate of T1 tumours
D. T3 tumours may be treated with radical cystectomy and urinary diversion
E. T3 tumours may be treated with radiotherapy alone

Q27 According to the TNM classification of bladder cancer:

A. T1 lesions have not invaded the lamina propria
B. T3a neoplasms have not invaded the perivesical fat
C. Ta tumours are confined to the bladder epithelium
D. Tumours invading the pelvic wall are stage T4b
E. A tumour that has penetrated the whole thickness of the muscle wall will be class-
ified T2

Q28 In the management of bladder calculi:

A. Cystoscopy is the most accurate means of diagnosis
B. The viewing lithotrite is particularly suitable for large and hard stones
C. The viewing lithotrite is used in such a way that its jaws face upwards
D. A Pfannenstiel incision is usually used when a suprapubic surgical procedure is
undertaken
E. Suby G solution may be used to prevent formation

Q29 In transurethral resection of the prostate (TURP):

A. The bladder neck is completely resected
B. The chips in the bladder are washed out by isotonic normal saline during the
operation
C. The chips may be evacuated by an Ellik's evacuator
D. The transurethral catheter is usually removed 24–48 hours after operation
E. Prostates larger than 90 g are particularly suitable for resection

Q30 Prostate specific antigen (PSA):

A. Is solely produced by the prostatic epithelial cells
B. Is a less sensitive serum marker for prostatic cancer than prostatic acid phosphatase
(PAP)
C. Serum levels greater than 1 ng/ml after radical prostatectomy are a sign of active
disease
D. Velocity is valuable in screening
E. Level may be elevated in benign prostatic hyperplasia

162

Q31 Benign prostatic hyperplasia (BPH):

A. Mainly occurs in the outer caudal zone of the prostate   F
B. Causes a downward displacement of the verumontanum
C. Consists of acini lined by one layer of epithelial cells
D. Is a recognised cause of vesicoureteric reflux
E. Commonly causes the serum prostate specific antigen (PSA) to be elevated above
    50 ng/ml   F

Q32 Pure seminoma:

A. Is associated with elevated serum levels of α-fetoprotein
B. Does not cause elevation of serum levels of hCG
C. Is radiosensitive
D. Invading the scrotal skin will be staged as T3b according to TNM classification
E. May present with backache

Q33 TURP is to be preferred to open prostatectomy as a treatment for benign prostatic hyperplasia in a patient with:

A. A prostate weighing about 110 g
B. Ankylosis of both hips
C. A small bladder diverticulum
D. A prostate weighing 45 g   T
E. Chronic obstructive airways disease T

Answers to Section 19

Q1
A. **True**
B. **True** – The affected testicle lies lower than the contralateral one
C. **True** – This can be performed during venography
D. **False** – An inguinal approach is usually adopted
E. **False**

Q2
A. **True**
B. **False** – They precipitate in acid urine
C. **True**
D. **False** – Infection is a contraindication for ESWL
E. **True**

Q3
A. **True**
B. **True**
C. **False**
D. **False**
E. **True**

Q4
A. **False** – It occurs in 2% of boys
B. **False** – It is commoner on the right side
C. **True** – Or LHRH
D. **False** – The malignancy risk is not significantly reduced by orchidopexy
E. **False** – Orchidopexy should be performed at the age of 1 year

Q5
A. **True**
B. **False** – These hydroceles often resolve within the first year, therefore surgery should be considered if they persist beyond the first year
C. **True** – This is true of very tense hydroceles
D. **True**
E. **True** – In Lord's procedure the sac is sutured to itself behind the testicle

Q6
A. **True**
B. **False** – This is contraindicated as it increases the risk of scrotal wall metastases
C. **True** – Cis-platinum, bleomycin and vinblastin are the main agents
D. **False** – Inguinal orchidectomy should be performed
E. **True**

163

Q7

A. **False**
B. **False**
C. **True** – Teratoma of the trophoblastic variety may do this
D. **False** – It is more likely to spread via the blood stream
E. **False** – Differentiated teratoma has the best prognosis

Q8

A. **False** – It has a segmental blood supply but there are no anastomoses
B. **False** – It is derived from the metanephros
C. **True** – However, this is not very reliable
D. **False** – Otherwise the transplanted kidney would not work
E. **True**

Q9

A. **True**
B. **False** – It crosses anterior to it
C. **False** – It is crossed anteriorly by the gonadal and ovarian vessels
D. **False** – It passes behind it
E. **True** – Therefore it should be mobilised from the medial side. The opposite is true in the abdomen

Q10

A. **True**
B. **False** – There is cellular swelling and hypercellularity due to the immigration of inflammatory cells
C. **True** – "Tubulitis"
D. **False** – The cortex is predominantly affected. Therefore at biopsy adequate sampling of the cortex is essential
E. **True** – The subendothelial space may contain plasma, fibrin deposits, etc.

Q11

A. **True** – This fascia provides a plane of cleavage to the surgeon and prevents the spread of malignancy
B. **False** – The main blood supply is through the superior vesical artery – a branch of the internal iliac artery
C. **True**
D. **False** – It relaxes
E. **False** – The interlacing fibres criss-cross over the bladder wall

Q12

A. **False** – The total body sodium is usually normal
B. **False** – Osmolality decreases due to dilution
C. **True** – Dilutional hyponatraemia ensues
D. **True**
E. **True**

Q13
A. **True**
B. **False** – Phase 1 continues to rise during the scan in obstructive uropathy until the kidney becomes non-functioning
C. **True**
D. **False** – Hypervascular blush may be demonstrated in renal tumours
E. **True**

Q14
A. **False** – This may cause red urine
B. **True**
C. **False** – This may cause red urine
D. **True**
E. **True**

Q15
A. **False** – Free ionic iodine is toxic. Therefore iodine atoms are attached to benzoic acid
B. **False** – This may occur in an obstructed kidney
C. **False**
D. **True**
E. **True** – However, such complications are rare (1/200 000)

Q16
A. **True**
B. **False** – DRw6-positive grafts do better
C. **False** – They have a beneficial effect
D. **True**
E. **True**

Q17
A. **True**
B. **False** – They are controlled by the D region
C. **False** – ABO compatibility is essential for all transplants
D. **False** – Matching at the B and DR loci is more important
E. **True**

Q18
A. **False** – Strangury is the painful desire to pass urine
B. **True**
C. **False** – Transurethral catheterisation may cause more damage and therefore should be avoided
D. **False** – Urgent surgical intervention is indicated
E. **True**

Q19
A. **True**
B. **False** – Haematuria is a late symptom. A lump in a wasted child is the usual presentation. Pain is often present
C. **False** – Stage V is assigned to bilateral lesions
D. **False** – Radiotherapy is not required in stage I, but should be given to stage III tumours
E. **False** – A 5 day course of actinomycin D is given prior to surgery. A course of vincristine is also given after surgical removal

Q20
A. **True** – Due to secretion of parahormone-like substance by the tumour
B. **True**
C. **True**
D. **True**
E. **False** – Secondary polycythaemia is a recognised complication

Q21
A. **True**
B. **False** – This is a recognised indication for ESWL
C. **True**
D. **True**
E. **True**

Q22
A. **False** – The left kidney is placed in the *right* iliac fossa so that the renal pelvis lies anteriorly
B. **True**
C. **False** – End-to-end anastomosis to the proximal end of the internal iliac artery is usual
D. **False** – This is true of hyperacute rejection
E. **True** – By employing a submucous tunnel
Note: See Figure 19.1

Q23
A. **False** – It is usually caused by ascending infection
B. **False** – The kidney is usually impalpable due to tenderness and spasm of overlying muscle
C. **True**
D. **True** – Children's kidneys are still developing
E. **True**

Q24
A. **True** – Due to stone fragments or blood clots
B. **True**
C. **True**
D. **True**
E. **False**

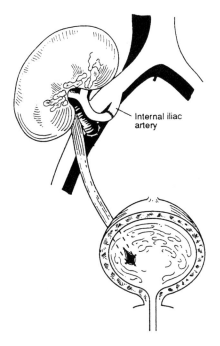

Internal iliac
artery

**Figure 19.1   Renal transplantation (anastomoses to the internal iliac artery, iliac vein and
bladder)**

Q25
A. **False**
B. **False**
C. **False**
D. **True**
E. **True** – Coagulation disorders are a contraindication

Q26
A. **True**
B. **True**
C. **False** – The recurrence rate can be reduced by, for example, thiotepa, mitomycin or
adriamycin
D. **True**
E. **True**

Q27
A. **False**
B. **True**
C. **True**
D. **True**
E. **False**
Note: See Figure 19.2

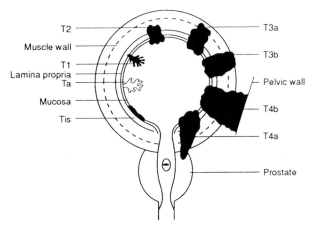

| T2 | | T3a |

Figure 19.2   TNM classification of bladder cancer

Q28
A. **True**
B. **False** – It is suitable for small and soft stones
C. **False** – The jaws face downwards in the opposite direction to a blind lithotrite
D. **True** – Surgery is indicated if transurethral removal is not possible (litholapaxy) or there is a coexisting pathology, e.g. diverticulum, enlarged prostate
E. **True**

Q29
A. **True**
B. **False** – Non-electrolytic solution must be used, e.g. 2% glycine
C. **True**
D. **True** – This is usually a three-way Foley catheter
E. **False** – Smaller prostates are more suitable for TURP

Q30
A. **True**
B. **False** – PSA is more sensitive than PAP
C. **True**
D. **True**
E. **True**

Q31
A. **False** – The inner cranial zone is usually affected
B. **True**
C. **False** – This is a feature of prostatic carcinoma. The acini are lined by two layers
D. **True**
E. **False** – Serum PSA levels may be elevated but not to this level

Q32
A. **False** – This has not been reported
B. **False** – Serum β-hCG is a feature in about 7.5% of cases
C. **True** – Radiotherapy is a primary treatment
D. **False** – It is staged as T4B
E. **True** – Due to retroperitoneal lymph node involvement

Q33
A. **False**
B. **False** – This prevents positioning for endoscopic surgery
C. **False** – Diverticulum does not necessarily require surgical treatment
D. **True**
E. **True**

20. Statistics and Screening

Q1   With reference to clinical trials:

A. In crossover designs, patients act as their own controls
B. The power of the trial equals the type I error
C. Type I error describes the probability of false positives
D. Type I error describes the possibility of rejecting a null hypothesis when it is in fact valid
E. The number of patients required for the trial depends on type I and II errors

Q2   In screening for colorectal cancer, the haemoccult test:

A. Gives a cancer detection rate of 3/1000
B. Gives a rate of false positives of 5%
C. False positive results may be caused by carrots
D. Utilises a peroxidase enzyme to increase sensitivity
E. If positive is an indication for colonoscopy

Q3   The incidence of colorectal cancer is increased in patients with:

A. Muir's syndrome
B. Peutz–Jegher's syndrome
C. Crohn's disease of the colon
D. Ureterosigmoidostomy
E. Gardner's syndrome

Q4   Audit:

A. Is derived from "audition"
B. Demands confidentiality for success
C. Should focus only on patient outcome
D. Is a strategy for identifying and punishing wrongdoers
E. Is valuable in validating routine procedures

Q5   Student's _t_ test:

A. Is a non-parametric test
B. Is appropriate if more than two means are compared
C. Gives a larger value of _t_, the smaller the value of _p_
D. Distribution is a normal distribution
E. Is not applicable to paired data

Answers to Section 20

Q1
A. **True**
B. **False** – It equals type II error
C. **True**
D. **False** – It describes the probability of accepting a null hypothesis when it is in fact invalid
E. **True** – And the minimal relevant difference

Q2
A. **True**
B. **False** – The false positive rate is 25%
C. **True** – Ferrous sulphate and red meat also cause false-positive results
D. **False** – A peroxidase inhibitor may be added
E. **True**

Q3
A. **True**
B. **True**
C. **True**
D. **True**
E. **True**

Q4
A. **True**
B. **True** – To both patients and clinical participants
C. **False** – Patient outcome measured in terms of morbidity, mortality or quality adjusted life years (QALYs) is important, but structure and process should also be part of the audit
D. **False** – It is primarily an educational exercise
E. **True**

Q5
A. **False** – It is a parametric test
B. **False**
C. **True** – And the stronger the evidence that the null hypothesis is untrue
D. **False** – It becomes normal at infinite degrees of freedom
E. **False** – The paired t test can be used

Part 2
Extended Matching Questions

Theme I
The Acute Abdomen

Options:

A. Acute cholecystitis
B. Perforated peptic ulcer
C. Acute embolic mesenteric ischaemia
D. Small bowel obstruction
E. Acute pancreatitis
F. Acute diverticulitis

For each of the patients described below, select the *single* most likely diagnosis from the list of options above. Each option may be used once, more than once or not at all.

Q1
A 62-year-old woman with a long-standing history of atrial fibrillation presents to the Accident and Emergency Department with a history of sudden onset of severe abdominal pain.

She has had a large bowel movement since the onset of pain and vomited once. No flatus has been passed since that time. Clinical examination reveals a mildly distended abdomen which is diffusely tender. She has tachycardia (120 bpm), Kussmaul breathing and hypotension (100/50 mmHg). Her Hb is 13 g/dl, WCC is 23 000/mm^3, serum amylase 500 units, serum potassium 5.8 mmol/l and creatinine 160 µmol/l. Abdominal and chest radiographs have no diagnostic features. Ten years ago she underwent an abdominal hysterectomy.

Q2
A 52-year-old man presents to the Accident and Emergency Department with a two-day history of severe epigastric pain of gradual onset radiating to the back and associated with nausea and vomiting.

Clinical examination reveals tachycardia (120 bpm), tachypnoea (38 rpm), hypotension (95/60 mmHg), a tender mass in the upper abdomen and a peri-umbilical ecchymosis.

Theme II
Endocrine Problems

Options:

A. Total gastrectomy
B. Calcitonin
C. Subtotal parathyroidectomy
D. Highly selective vagotomy
E. Total thyroidectomy
F. Pancreatectomy

For each of the patients described below, select the *single* most likely treatment from the list of options above. Each option may be used once, more than once or not at all.

Q3
A 39-year-old sister of a patient with multiple endocrine neoplasia type I (Werner's syndrome) is found on biochemical screening to have elevated serum calcium, parathyroid hormone and gastrin. She has an abnormal response to secretin stimulation.

Q4
A 35-year-old man on haemodialysis complains of bone pain and pruritus.

Serum biochemistry reveals hypocalcaemia, hyperphosphataemia and an elevated serum PTH level (four times normal). His symptoms persist despite treatment with vitamin D, oral calcium supplements, phosphate-binding antacids and high-calcium dialysis bath.

Theme III
Multiple Trauma

Options:

A. Haemothorax
B. Cardiac tamponade
C. Ruptured spleen
D. Flail chest
E. Tension pneumothorax
F. Aortic rupture

For each of the patients described below, select the most likely *single* diagnosis from the list of options above. Each option may be used once, more than once or not at all.

Q5

A 24-year-old man is brought into the Accident and Emergency Department following a road traffic accident.

He is conscious. He has tachypnoea (40 rpm), tachycardia (130 bpm) and distended neck veins. His systemic BP is 85/40 mmHg. His heart sounds are greatly diminished. A chest radiograph shows three fractured ribs (ribs 5, 6 and 7) on the left side and a small pneumothorax. A left chest drain and central venous catheter are inserted. The CVP is 20 cm. The BP is 90/50 mmHg after 2 litres of colloids infusion. The ECG shows reduced voltage in QRS complexes.

Q6

A 50-year-old woman is brought into the Accident and Emergency Department following a road traffic accident.

She is conscious with adequate airway. The GCS is 15. She is tachypnoeic (30 rpm). Her pulse is 150 bpm and reduced in volume. The distal pulses are present. Her BP is 85/45 mmHg. The chest radiograph shows multiple rib fractures on the left side (ribs 7, 8 and 9) and a 20% pneumothorax. A left chest drain is inserted (100 ml of blood is drained). The CVP is −2 cm. Analysis of the diagnostic peritoneal lavage (DPL) fluid reveals a WCC of 1000/mm^3 and an amylase level of 400 units. She remains hypotensive (BP 90/55 mmHg) despite the infusion of 5 units of colloids and 4 units of blood.

Theme IV
Pancreatic and Hepatobiliary Disease

Options:

A. Ascending cholangitis
B. Primary biliary cirrhosis
C. Cholangiocarcinoma
D. Carcinoma of the pancreatic head
E. Mirizzi's syndrome
F. A stone in the common bile duct (CBD)

For each of the patients described below, select the most likely *single* diagnosis from the list of options above. Each option may be used once, more than once or not at all.

Q7

A 67-year-old woman presents with backache and weight loss.

Clinical examination shows jaundice, wasting and a palpable mass in the right upper quadrant. FBC reveals anaemia. Liver function tests show raised liver enzymes (AST 230 U/l, ALT 215 U/l, ALP 1100 U/l), jaundice (bilirubin 190 µmol/l) and low albumin. Her serum amylase and glucose are normal.

Q8

A 50-year-old man presents with intermittent upper abdominal pain and jaundice four weeks after laparoscopic cholecystectomy for gallstones.

Clinical examination shows jaundice only. Liver function tests suggest obstructive jaundice. The CBD on ultrasonography is 15 mm in diameter.

Theme V
Colorectal Cancer

Options:

A. Hartmann's procedure
B. 5-Fluorouracil infusion
C. Anterior resection of the rectum
D. Abdominoperineal (AP) resection of the rectum
E. Defunctioning loop ileostomy
F. Radical radiotherapy

For each of the patients described below, select the *single* most likely treatment from the list of options above. Each option may be used once, more than once or not at all.

Q9

A 49-year-old man presents to the Accident and Emergency Department with rectal bleeding and altered bowel habits.

Rigid sigmoidoscopy demonstrates a stenosing tumour at the rectosigmoid junction; a biopsy is taken. Histological examination confirms the presence of a moderately differentiated colorectal carcinoma. Abdominal ultrasonography reveals multiple metastases in both lobes of the liver. A barium enema shows no other abnormality in the colon. Computed tomography suggests that the primary tumour is operable and confirms hepatic metastases.

Q10

A 57-year-old woman presents with rectovaginal fistula two weeks after anterior resection of the rectum for Dukes B carcinoma.

Theme VI
Colorectal Disease

Options:

A. Colorectal carcinoma
B. Ulcerative colitis
C. Crohn's disease
D. Colonic angiodysplasia
E. Diverticulitis
F. Ischaemic colitis

For each of the patients described below, select the *single* most likely diagnosis from the list of options above. Each option may be used once, more than once or not at all.

Q11

A 50-year-old woman is brought into the Accident and Emergency Department with profuse dark red rectal bleeding.

She is conscious. On examination she has a tachycardia of 120 bpm. Her BP is 90/60 mmHg. Following adequate resuscitation with colloids, crystalloids and blood, a radioisotope-labelled red blood cell scan is performed. The scan is positive in the right colon. The patient remains haemodynamically stable after initial resuscitation. A subsequent barium enema does not show any abnormality.

Q12

A 60-year-old man presents with a three-day history of pain in the left iliac fossa (LIF), blood-stained diarrhoea and fever.

Clinical examination demonstrates a tender mass in the LIF, pyrexia (38.5°C) and tachycardia (110 bpm). He has had several episodes of pain in the LIF over the past two years.

Theme VII
Thyroid Disease

Options:

A. Papillary carcinoma
B. Follicular adenoma
C. Lymphoma
D. Follicular carcinoma
E. Anaplastic carcinoma
F. Medullary thyroid carcinoma (MTC)

For each of the patients described below, select the most likely *single* diagnosis from the list of options above. Each option may be used once, more than once or not at all.

Q13

A 14-year-old girl presents to the Surgical Outpatient Department with a neck swelling.

Clinical examination shows a 3 cm solid lump in the left thyroid lobe and two enlarged cervical lymph nodes lateral to the thyroid mass. Ultrasonography confirms the solid nature of the thyroid nodule. FNA biopsy of the thyroid nodule reveals malignant cells with a vesicular appearance to the nuclei. The nodule is cold on radioisotope scanning.

Q14

A 25-year-old man presents with a thyroid swelling. He also complains of diarrhoea and episodic flushing.

Clinical examination reveals a 2.5 cm solid nodule in the right thyroid lobe and no other abnormality. He has been taking nifedipine (20 mg daily) for recently diagnosed hypertension. His sister suffers from Cushing's syndrome. Ultrasound confirms the solid nature of the thyroid nodule and FNAB demonstrates malignant cells.

Theme VIII
Endocrine and Electrolyte Disturbance

Options:

A. Secondary hyperaldosteronism
B. A unilateral adenoma of the adrenal cortex
C. Addison's disease
D. Phaeochromocytoma
E. Pituitary Cushing's syndrome
F. Adrenocortical carcinoma

For each of the patients described below, select the most likely *single* diagnosis from the list of options above. Each option may be used once, more than once or not at all.

Q15

A 37-year-old man presents with muscle weakness and polyuria.

Clinical examination reveals hypertension (BP 170/110 mmHg). Biochemical analysis reveals hypokalaemia (2.6 mmol/l), hypernatraemia (150 mmol/l) and metabolic alkalosis. The serum aldosterone is elevated and plasma renin activity is undetectable. The plasma total cortisol is normal.

Q16

A 30-year-old woman presents with diabetes, hypertension and backache.

Biochemical analysis reveals hypokalaemia (2.8 mmol/l), raised plasma total cortisol and raised plasma ACTH. The high-dose dexamethasone suppression test is positive.

Answers

1. (C) The sudden onset of the pain, atrial fibrillation and bowel opening support this diagnosis. The Kussmaul breathing and hyperkalaemia may be due to associated metabolic acidosis. Further investigations include arterial blood gas analysis and mesenteric angiography.

2. (E) The gradual onset of pain, the radiation to the back, the periumbilical ecchymosis (Cullen's sign) and the hypoxemia make acute pancreatitis most likely.

3. (C) Hyperparathyroidism should be treated first. Serum gastrin may decline after correcting serum calcium. If gastrin levels remain high, treatment of the Zollinger–Ellison component of the syndrome should be considered.

4. (C) The patient has secondary hyperparathyroidism refractory to conservative management.

5. (B)

6. (C) Hypotension, tachycardia and low CVP suggest hypovolaemia. Multiple rib fractures on the left side and positive DPL support the diagnosis of splenic rupture.

7. (D) Backache, obstructive jaundice, palpable gall bladder and weight loss are compatible with the diagnosis of pancreatic cancer.

8. (F) The ERCP may reveal a filling defect in the CBD. The incidence of CBD injuries and strictures is higher after laparoscopic cholecystectomy.

9. (C) Surgical resection of the primary lesion remains the best form of palliation in the presence of distant metastases. The patient may require further adjuvant chemotherapy and radiotherapy.

10. (E)

11. (D)

12. (E) This patient should be treated conservatively with IV fluids and antimicrobials. The mass in the LIF is most likely to be inflammatory in nature and should be investigated with ultrasonography and/or CT. A barium enema should be arranged when the acute presentation settles.

13. (A) The presence of regional lymphadenopathy, the age of the patient and the characteristic vesicular appearance of the nuclei support the diagnosis of papillary carcinoma. The surgical treatment consists of total thyroidectomy and removal of enlarged lymph nodes.

14. (F) The recently diagnosed hypertension may be due to phaeochromocytoma; diarrhoea and episodic flushing are associated with MTC. The latter is the only thyroid tumour associated with Cushing's syndrome. The most likely diagnosis is multiple endocrine neoplasia (MEN) – type IIa.

15. (B) In secondary hyperaldosteronism, the plasma renin activity is usually elevated. The most likely diagnosis is Conn's syndrome. The commonest cause is a solitary adrenal adenoma (85%). MRI or CT confirms the diagnosis in 80% of cases.

16. (E) The elevated serum ACTH and positive high-dose dexamethasone suppression test support the diagnosis of pituitary Cushing's syndrome. The backache may be due to osteoporosis. Hypertension and diabetes are recognised manifestations of the syndrome.